THE DICTIONARY OF MINERALS

An invaluable reference book giving full, up-to-date information on the complete range of minerals and mineral therapy.

THE DICTIONARY OF MINERALS

The complete guide to minerals and mineral therapy

Compiled and written by
LEONARD MERVYN
B.Sc., Ph.D., C.Chem., F.R.S.C.
Member of the New York Academy of Sciences

THORSONS PUBLISHING GROUP
Wellingborough · New York

First published 1985

Published in the UK by Thorsons Publishers Ltd.,
Denington Estate, Wellingborough, Northamptonshire NN8 2RQ,
and in the USA by Thorsons Publishers Inc.,
377 Park Avenue South, New York, NY 10016

DEDICATION

This book is dedicated to my wife's parents,
Sarah Brown and William (Bud) Brown,
with gratitude and affection.

British Library Cataloguing in Publication Data

Mervyn, Leonard
  The dictionary of minerals: the complete
  guide to minerals and mineral therapy.
  1. Minerals in the body
  I. Title
  612'.01524   QP533

ISBN 0-7225-1172-8

Printed and bound in Great Britain

INTRODUCTION

Whilst most people are aware of the need for vitamins in their diets, mainly because of much publicity in the popular press during the last few years, there appears to be little knowledge on those equally important nutrients the minerals. Mention minerals to the average person and they will immediately think of iron for the blood and calcium for the bones and leave it at that. Any woman who has been pregnant will almost certainly have been prescribed iron and calcium to be taken during her pregnancy because these two minerals are known to be essential for the growing foetus and they also represent those most likely to be deficient in her diet. What is being gradually realized is that perhaps lack of other minerals may also represent a risk to the pregnant mother and we should look beyond iron and calcium.

Minerals are unique amongst dietary nutrients because they are relatively difficult to absorb from the food eaten. Under normal circumstances the digestion products of fats, carbohydrates and proteins are efficiently absorbed along with vitamins and we usually assume near 100 per cent assimilation. Most minerals however average only between 10 and 15 per cent absorption. The exceptions are the simple ions like sodium, potassium and chloride which are virtually completely absorbed. The relatively poor level of absorption of the other minerals is probably due to (a) only a short length of intestine is available for absorption, and (b) the intestinal tract exerts some control over the amount of minerals absorbed. This in turn depends upon the body status of the minerals.

Although minerals, unlike vitamins, cannot be destroyed, they can be removed by the processing and refining of foodstuffs. They can also be rendered insoluble and unavailable for absorption by other constituents of the diet. All minerals are ultimately obtained from the soil in which plants grow so any deficiency there will reflect in the mineral content of those plants. In other words, eating plant foods is no guarantee that the full mineral complement is present. When we consider all these obstacles culminating in a pretty inefficient rate of absorption, perhaps it is not surprising that many researchers are looking more closely at the true level of intake of the essential minerals from today's diets.

Like vitamins, our needs for individual minerals cover a wide range of intakes required for health. At one end of the scale are calcium, phosphorus and magnesium where the daily quantity required is measured in hundreds of milligrams; at the oother end are iodine, selenium and chromium where dietary needs are measured in hundreds of micrograms. Yet the manifestations of deficiency of the so-called trace elements can be just as damaging to the health as a deficiency in those of the gross or macro-elements. In the past, research has tended to be directed towards the macro-elements but now, long overdue, we are just beginning to look into the importance of those essential minerals needed only in tiny amounts. The tragedy is that the factors mentioned above that can affect our eventual assimilation of minerals are more likely to apply to the trace elements because they are present in such small concentration anyway. Iron and calcium are used to fortify white flour but no one bothers to replace all the other minerals removed by the refining process to produce it.

We have seen over the past thirty years or so how some vitamins, taken in high potency far beyond their requirements in a vitamin function, can exert an actual therapeutic effect in some disorders. There does not seem to be a parallel case for minerals. In other words, minerals need only be taken when there is a deficiency of them. There are very good reasons for this. In the case of the gross elements excessive amounts are wasteful since the body will simply reject what it does not want. Remember that it is the minerals not absorbed that cause problems in the gastro-intestinal tract — iron is a good example.

As far as the trace minerals are concerned, there is in some of them a fairly narrow gap between the amount required for health and that which will produce toxic effects. Hence if you wish to take supplementary minerals in the absence of professional guidance, ensure that the dosage taken is that suggested on the pack. There is little point in taking more.

A

---

acid-base balance, the balance between the amount of carbonic acid and bicarbonate base in the blood which must be maintained at a constant ratio of 1 to 20 to ensure the pH of the blood is kept between 7.35 and 7.45. In the healthy individual the blood is maintained within this narrow range of alkalinity. This pH value depends upon two mechanisms: the rate of excretion of carbonic acid (i.e. aqueous carbon dioxide) through the lungs in the expired air; and the ability of the kidneys to excrete either an acid or alkaline urine. When the lungs and kidneys are diseased these mechanisms may no longer function efficiently and an acidosis (excess acid) or alkalosis (excess alkali or base) results.

Dietary aspects of acid-base balance are less important than metabolic defects but can still influence the acidity or alkalinity of the body and hence that of the urine. For example, a rabbit has a diet consisting mainly of green and other vegetables and normally excretes an alkaline urine. A dog, which is carnivorous or omnivorous, excretes an acid urine. Vegetarian human beings usually excrete a neutral or slightly alkaline urine. Omnivorous human beings will excrete a slightly acid urine; large meat eaters will excrete a more acid urine. The reason is because meat protein is high in sulphur which the body converts to sulphuric acid before excretion in the urine. The high phosphorus content of meat ends up as phosphoric acid which also contributes to the acidity of the urine.

Dietary acids are organic acids present in fruit, vegetables and yogurt. Contrary to popular belief they do not produce acid reactions within the body (acidosis) and are in fact alkali-forming. Examples of such acids in the diet are:

1. citric acid (citrus fruits, pineapple, tomato, most summer fruits).

Citric acid is oxidized by the body in its normal energy production cycle.

2.   malic acid (apples, plums, tomatoes). Malic acid is oxidized by the body in its normal energy production cycle.

3.   benzoic acid (cranberry, bilberry). Benzoic acid is readily excreted by the kidney (after combination with the amino acid glycine) as hippuric acid.

4.   tartaric acid (grapes). This acid is hardly absorbed so does not contribute to the acid-base balance of the body.

5.   oxalic acid (strawberries, green tomatoes, rhubarb, spinach). Oxalic acid can combine with calcium to form insoluble calcium oxalate so it is not absorbed. However, excess oxalic acid can immobilize calcium and other minerals to an extent that may cause mild deficiency. Any oxalic acid absorbed is readily oxidized by existing metabolic processes.

6.   lactic acid (yogurt). Is metabolized by the same body processes that dispose of lactic acid produced from glucose. Foods are either acid-producing or alkali-producing, depending upon how the body metabolizes them. It is believed by some that an excess of acid-producing foods in the diet is a factor in inducing arthritis. Treatment of the condition is therefore aimed at switching to an alkali-producing diet.

Acid-forming foods are: meats of all kinds (with the exception of horse); poultry; fish and all sea foods; lentils; onions; brazil nuts; peanuts; walnuts; pearl barley; bread, all types of wheat and other cereal flours; all types of pasta; oatflakes; rice; semolina; tapioca; cocoa powder; chocolate; eggs; all cheeses.

Alkali-forming foods are: all fruits; all fruit juices; all vegetables (with the exception of lentils and onions); all vegetable juices; honey; molasses; cream; fresh milk of all types and treated milks (buttermilk, evaporated, condensed, dried); horseflesh; wine.

---

acid bismuth sodium tartrate,   provides 38-44mg bismuth in each 100mg. Dose is 120-300mg. Has been employed in conjunction with the enzyme pepsin, for digestive disorders. For toxic effects *see* bismuth.

---

acidosis,   a condition in which the acidity of the body fluids and tissue is abnormally high, producing a low pH. Induced by a failure of the acid-base balance mechanism.

Lactic acidosis is due to:

1.   accumulation of large amounts of lactic acid in the blood after severe muscular exercise. Rapid breathing during the recovery phase helps to

restore the acid-base balance by removing excess carbon dioxide through the lungs.

2. inadequate oxygenation of the tissues in certain diseases (e.g. heart failure);

3. loss of sodium, potassium and ketone bodies in the urine of those suffering from diabetes;

4. some liver diseases;

5. intravenous infusions of fructose.

Metabolic acidosis may be due to:

1. kidney failure;

2. lactic acidosis;

3. poisons such as ethylene glycol, salicylates;

4. acetoacetic acid that accumulates in the blood of diabetics;

5. excessive loss of alkali from the intestinal tract, as in diarrhoea;

6. ingestion of ammonium chloride.

Symptoms of acidosis include: increased depth and frequency of respiration; vague lassitude; nausea; vomiting. Apart from acidosis induced by severe muscular exertion, all other causes need medical management.

---

acne,   inflammation of the hair and sweat glands. Has been treated with zinc at a supplementary dose of 20mg of the element daily. Appears to function by acting as an anti-inflammatory agent — reducing the irritation and removing the characteristic red blotches that often accompany the pimples — by restoring the hormone balance that may be upset at puberty, which is the period of life at which the condition is most prevalent. Some evidence of low body zinc levels at puberty.

---

acrodermatitis enteropathica,   a rare inherited disorder characterized by a psoriatic dermatitis, hair loss, infections of the nails, growth retardation and diarrhoea. Once fatal, it is now known to be due to malabsorption of zinc leading to low levels in the blood plasma. Complete remission is obtained with daily doses of 35-150mg zinc sulphate, providing 8-34mg zinc.

---

aldosterone,   a steroid hormone, elaborated by the adrenal cortex, that acts upon the kidney to regulate water balance by causing sodium retention and potassium loss. Used medically to treat deficient production and in the treatment of shock. Overproduction of aldosterone leads to excessive blood and tissue levels of sodium and loss of potassium, causing water retention and eventually high blood pressure. One class of diuretic drugs acts by inhibiting the action of aldosterone. *See* diuretic drugs.

---

alkalosis, a condition in which the alkalinity of body fluids and tissue is abnormally high, producing a high pH. It is due to failure of the mechanisms that maintain a normal acid-base balance. It may be associated with certain diuretic therapy; loss of acid through persistent vomiting; excessive sodium bicarbonate intake; deep breathing not associated with physical exercise. Symptoms of alkalosis are muscular weakness or cramp.

Apart from that produced by abnormally deep breathing, alkalosis usually requires medical management.

---

aluminium, chemical symbol A1. Atomic weight 27.0. Third most abundant element in the earth's crust at a level of 8.8g per 100g. Occurs mainly in combination with silica (aluminium silicates) and as aluminium oxide.

Present in trace amounts in plants, animals and man but it does not appear to act as an essential element.

Storage in the body is in the lungs, liver, thyroid and brain. Later most of the dietary aluminium is excreted.

In the diet aluminium may be supplied from aluminium cooking pots used to cook acid-containing foods or liquids; some baking powders; food additives. Aluminium-containing preparations are widely used as antacids representing another source. Water used in dialysing solutions for those on kidney dialysis may also contribute aluminium.

Functions of aluminium in the body are not known but it is used in medicine:

1. as an antacid, to relieve the pain in gastric and duodenal ulcers and in reflux oesophagitis (heartburn) by neutralizing hydrochloric acid in the gastric secretions. Aluminium salts used for this purpose include: (a) aluminium glycinate; (b) aluminium hydroxide; (c) aluminium phosphate; (d) aluminium sodium silicate.

2. as an astringent to form a superficial protective layer over damaged skin and mucous membrances. Preparations include: (a) aluminium potassium sulphate (alum); (b) aluminium acetotartrate; (c) aluminium chloride; (d) aluminium chlorohydrate; (e) aluminium formate;

(f) aluminium subacetate; (g) aluminium sulphate; (h) ammonia alum.
3. to reduce phosphate absorption in those with chronic kidney failure;
4. to treat disorders of the mouth. Preparations include aluminium
lactate. The astringent properties of aluminium salts are also utilized in
cosmetic preparations and in deodorants.

Food additives containing aluminium include aluminium metal;
aluminium calcium silicate; aluminium potassium sulphate; aluminium
sodium silicate.

Toxic effects of aluminium on the skin include contact dermatitis and
irritation in sensitive people. Internally, the mineral can cause phosphate
depletion and skeletal demineralization resembling osteomalacia in those
undergoing kidney dialysis; brain dysfunction in those undergoing kidney
dialysis; brain degeneration characteristic of some types of senile dementia;
slow learning in the young; epileptic-type fits in experimental animals;
exacerbation of osteoporosis.

Levels of 12 μg aluminium per g brain tissue that give rise to brain
deterioration in experimental animals are the same as those found in the
brains of human beings who suffered from Alzheimer's disease or senile
dementia. This suggests that aluminium may be a factor in these diseases
of human beings.

---

aluminium calcium silicate, a food additive also known as calcium
aluminium silicate; calcium aluminosilicate; calcium silicoaluminate.
Functions as an anti-caking agent. Provides 9.9mg aluminium; 29.2mg
calcium; 20.5mg silica per 100mg. No limit on acceptable daily intake.
A permitted miscellaneous additive.

---

aluminium potassium sulphate, a food additive also known as
potassium aluminium sulphate; alum; potash alum. Functions as a firming
agent restricted to glacé cherries. Provides 5.7mg aluminium; 8.24mg
potassium; 13.5mg sulphur per 100mg. No acceptable daily intake allocated
yet.

---

aluminium sodium silicate, a food additive also known as sodium
aluminium silicate; sodium aluminosilicate; sodium silicoaluminate.
Functions as an anti-caking agent and can be used in all foods. Provides
15.4mg aluminium; 44.6mg potassium; 8.0mg silica per 100mg. No limit

on acceptable daily intake. A permitted miscellaneous additive.

amino-acid chelates, minerals that are organically bound to amino acids. They may occur as such in foods or they can be produced from mineral salts within the small intestine from amino acids that are formed from the normal digestion of protein. It is also possible to produce amino-acid chelates by mimicking the natural process under controlled laboratory conditions. Soy or other protein that is broken down by enzymes supplies the amino acids required; coupling with the mineral is carried out by adjusting the pH of the mixture and creating the ideal conditions for specific mineral chelates. Amino-acid chelates may also be stabilized by buffering them to ensure they survive the acid/alkali changes of the digestive tract.

Many studies indicate that amino-acid chelation of minerals is a natural process that increases the rate and extent of absorption of the mineral compared with other mineral preparations; enhances the retention of the minerals; improves the extent of utilization of the minerals; protects the mineral against precipitating factors like phosphate, oxalate and phytic acid; reduces the side-effects of unabsorbed mineral on the gastrointestinal system.

ammonium chloride, a food additive that is used in yeast food and as a flavour. Provides 67.0mg chloride per 100mg. No limit on acceptable daily intake. Is a miscellaneous additive.

Used in medicine to acidify the urine when infection of the urinary tract is present; aid the excretion of certain drugs; increase the diuretic effect of mercurials; hasten lead excretion; supply chloride in chloride replacement therapy; act as an expectorant in cough mixtures.

ammonium dihydrogen orthophosphate, a food additive also known as ammonium phosphate, monobasic. Functions as additive to yeast food; as an emulsifying salt; as a buffer. Provides 27.0mg phosphorus per 100mg. Acceptable daily intake is up to 70mg phosphorus per kg body weight when calcium intake is normal. Permitted in certain cheeses and as a miscellaneous additive.

ammonium iodide, provides 87.6µg iodine in 100µg iodide. Used in a similar manner to potassium iodide.

Daily dose is from 120-400mg for pre-operative and expectorant use. As a supplement 200-1200µg per day is sufficient. Toxicity as for potassium iodide.

---

ammonium phosphate, dibasic, a food additive also known as diAmmonium hydrogen orthophosphate. Functions as additive to yeast food; as an emulsifying salt; as a buffer. Provides 23.5mg phosphorus per 100mg. Acceptable daily intake is up to 70mg phosphorus per kg body weight when calcium intake is normal. Permitted in certain cheeses; in certain wines; as a miscellaneous additive.

---

ammonium polyphosphates, food additives permitted in some cheeses and as miscellaneous additives. Acceptable daily intake is up to 70mg phosphorus per kg body weight when calcium intake is normal. Used as emulsifying salts; curing acids; to bind and retain water in meats and poultry.

---

ammonium sulphate, food additive that functions as a yeast food. Provides 24.2mg sulphur per 100mg. Permitted in certain wines and as a miscellaneous additive. Acceptable daily intake not determined.

---

anaemia, the iron-deficiency type which is the most common may be caused by:
1. low dietary intakes of iron because of poor diet;
2. poor absorption of dietary iron;
3. inefficient incorporation into haemoglobin;
4. pregnancy, because of the demands of the growing foetus for iron;
5. lactation, because of loss of iron through breast milk;
6. losses of iron being greater than dietary absorption, as in menstruation;
in gastric and duodenal ulcers; in haemorrhoids (piles); in some drug treatments, e.g. aspirin.

A rare type of anaemia where iron is adequate may be due to low intakes of copper which is needed for incorporation of iron into haemoglobin. Most iron-deficiency anaemias respond to iron supplementation (up to

75mg elemental iron daily), but small amounts of copper (up to 2mg daily) and vitamin C (100mg with each iron dose) will help the iron to be absorbed and utilized more efficiently. If the deficiency is due to malabsorption or greatly increased losses, professional help is needed to treat the underlying cause. *See also* iron.

anorexia nervosa,   a disorder characterized by a marked anxiety about body weight and weight gain resulting in abnormal patterns of handling food, serious weight loss and cessation of periods in women. The usual treatment is psychotherapy, but there is one case on record where zinc supplementation was successful in restoring loss of taste, increase in weight and a return to normal eating habits. Treatment consisted of 15mg zinc (as zinc sulphate) three times daily with meals. A good response was apparent after two weeks but further progress was continued only after the dose was increased to 50mg zinc (as zinc sulphate) three times daily. The main indications of zinc deficiency were loss of taste and loss of smell and these were used throughout to monitor zinc status of the female.

apples,   a low sodium food that supplies useful amounts of potassium and iron with only small quantities of the other minerals.

Eating variety supplies (in mg per 100g): sodium 2; potassium 120; calcium 4; magnesium 5; phosphorus 8; iron 0.3; copper 0.04; zinc 0.1; sulphur 6; chloride 1.

Cooking variety supplies (in mg per 100g), for raw, baked and stewed respectively: sodium 2, 2, 2; potassium 120, 130, 100; calcium 4, 4, 3; magnesium 3, 3, 3; phosphorus 16, 17, 14; iron 0.3, 0.3, 0.3; copper 0.09, 0.09, 0.08; zinc 0.1, 0.1, 0.1; sulphur 3, 3, 3; chloride 5, 5, 4.

apricots,   a low sodium food that is an excellent source of potassium, calcium, magnesium, iron and copper. The dried variety is even richer in these minerals. Stewing with sugars reduces the mineral content slightly because of dilution.

Dried, raw supplies (in mg per 100g): sodium 56; potassium 1880; calcium 92; magnesium 65; phosphorus 120; iron 4.1; copper 0.27; zinc 0.2; sulphur 160; chloride 35.

Stewed (without stones), without sugar and with sugar respectively: sodium 21, 20; potassium 700, 670; calcium 34, 33; magnesium 24, 23;

phosphorus 44, 43; iron 1.5, 1.5; copper 0.1, 0.1; zinc 0.1, 0.1; sulphur 59, 57; chloride 13, 12.

---

arrowroot, a poor source of most minerals but supplies some iron and copper. Minerals present are (in mg per 100g): sodium 5; potassium 18; calcium 7; magnesium 8; phosphorus 27; iron 2.0; copper 0.22; sulphur 2; chloride 7.

---

arsenic, chemical symbol As. Atomic weight 74.9. Abundance in the earth's crust is 0.0005 per cent. Occurs in nature as the free metal and in combination with other metals.

Small amounts present in most body tissues as a result of dietary intakes within the range 0.4-3.9mg per day. Most dietary arsenic ends up in the liver and muscle which can have concentrations up to 49 and 195 μg per 100g respectively. Excretion is fairly rapid, so toxic levels from the diet do not build up.

The richest food sources of arsenic are shellfish. Some meats contain organic arsenic which was originally added to the animals' feeds. Poultry and pigs are given traces of arsenic to improve growth. Arsenic compounds are used as insecticides which find their way to the soil and hence to plants which, when eaten, represent another dietary source. Water, too, contributes arsenic to the diet.

Traces of arsenic appear to be necessary for the health of animals but no specific functions have been assigned to the mineral. It is likely that it is also an essential trace mineral for man but such minute amounts are needed that a deficiency is highly unlikely.

Food and drink levels of arsenic are limited by law. Beverages may not contain more than 0.5mg per litre. Dried herbs may not contain more than 5.0mg per kg. Brewer's yeast is limited to less than 5.0mg per kg. WHO recommends that drinking water should not exceed 50 μg per litre.

Excessive intakes of arsenic can be fatal. Acute intoxication is indicated by severe gastric pain; vomiting; profuse watery diarrhoea; protein excretion in the urine; numbness and tingling in the hands and feet; intense thirst; muscular cramps. Eventually nerve complaints, kidney disease and brain damage result.

Chronic poisoning is characterized by oedema of the face and eyelids; generalized itching; sore mouth; inflammation of the eyes and nasal membranes; loss of appetite; nausea; vomiting; diarrhoea. Continued administration for long periods leads to dryness of the skin, dermatitis, pigmentation and hardness. Loss of hair and nails usually follows. Late symtoms include anaemia, cirrhosis of the liver; jaundice, neuritis.

Prolonged administration of sublethal amounts of arsenic may lead to cancer of the skin and lungs. Lethal intake can be as low as 100mg arsenic trioxide if taken in one dose.

Therapy with arsenic at oral doses of 1-5mg arsenic trioxide was originally used for syphilis. Externally it has been used in treating dermatitis, eczema and syphilitic skin diseases. The therapeutic use of inorganic arsenic compounds is no longer recommended.

---

arthritis, *Rheumatoid*, inflammation of the joints. *Osteo*, degenerative joint disease characterized by calcified out-growths from cartilage. Both types have been reported as responding favourably to calcium supplement-ation at intakes between 500 and 1500mg daily. Reasons are not known, but even the calcified out-growths of osteo-arthritis, due to a high local concentration of the mineral, may disappear when low calcium levels elsewhere are remedied. Such low levels may originate in the bone reserves, as in osteoporosis, which is associated with some cases of arthritis.

Localized copper deficiencies may also be a factor in arthritic conditions, particularly the rheumatoid type. Copper bangles may contribute copper through the skin (*see* copper bangles). Some oral copper complexes, e.g those with aspirin, also appear to have an anti-inflammatory action greater than the aspirin itself. Organic forms of copper were more efficient than copper salts in relieving arthritic symptoms in experimental studies on animals.

---

artichoke, a low sodium food that supplies useful quantities of potassium, calcium and magnesium. When boiled provides the following minerals (in mg per 100g): sodium 6-15; potassium 140-330; calcium 19-44; magnesium 12-27; phosphorus 17-40; iron 0.2-0.5; copper 0.04-0.09; sulphur 7-16; chloride 36-84.

---

asparagus, virtually devoid of sodium, but supplies good intakes of potassium. When boiled provides mineral levels in the following ranges (in mg per 100g): sodium 1-2; potassium 120-240; calcium 13-26; magnesium 5-10; phosphorus 42-85; iron 0.5-0.9; copper 0.1-0.2; zinc

0.1-0.3; sulphur 23-47; chloride 16-31.

---

aubergine, a low sodium food that is a good source of potassium with only small quantities of other minerals. As raw provides (in mg per 100g): sodium 3; potassium 240; calcium 10; magnesium 10; phosphorus 12; iron 0.4; copper 0.08; sulphur 9; chloride 61.

---

avocado pears, a low sodium food that is a very good source of potassium, but also supplies useful intakes of iron and magnesium. Other minerals are low in concentration. Minerals present are (in mg per 100g): sodium 2; potassium 400; calcium 15; magnesium 29; phosphorus 31; iron 1.5; copper 0.21; sulphur 19; chloride 6.

B

---

bacon, high sodium content, introduced during curing process, but also a very good source of potassium, magnesium, phosphorus, iron, copper, zinc and sulphur. High chloride content due to addition during processing.

Minerals present (in mg per 100g) for all cooked varieties, ranging from: sodium 1910-2140; potassium 300-480; calcium 9-13; magnesium 20-31; phosphorus 170-260; iron 1.3-1.4; copper 0.12-0.17; zinc 2.6-3.2; sulphur 280-310; chloride 2970-3290.

---

baked beans, good source of potassium but more sodium is present because of addition before canning. Useful iron, copper, zinc and sulphur levels. Contains mineral levels (in mg per 100g) of: sodium 480; potassium 300; calcium 45; magnesium 31; phosphorus 91; iron 1.4; copper 0.21; zinc 0.7; sulphur 43; chloride 800.

---

baker's yeast, rich source of potassium, phosphorus, iron, copper and zinc, plus chromium and selenium. All contents are increased over threefold in the dried variety.

Fresh, compressed variety contains the following minerals (in mg per 100g): sodium 16; potassium 610; calcium 25; magnesium 59; phosphorus 390; iron 5.0; copper 1.6; zinc 2.6.

Dried variety (in mg per 100g) contains: sodium 50; potassium 2000; calcium 80; magnesium 230; phosphorus 1290; iron 20.0; copper 5.0; zinc 8.0.

---

banana, virtually sodium free with a very good level of potassium. Other minerals are present but in low concentration. Edible part only (in mg per 100g) contains: sodium 1; potassium 350; calcium 7; magnesium 42; phosphorus 28; iron 0.4; copper 0.16; zinc 0.2; sulphur 13; chloride 79.

Barcelona nuts, practically devoid of sodium but rich in potassium, calcium, magnesium, phosphorus, iron, copper, zinc and sulphur. One of the better sources of non-dairy calcium. Mineral quantities present (in mg per 100g) are: sodium 2; potassium 760; calcium 180; magnesium 410; phosphorus 590; iron 2.8; copper 1.10; zinc 4.2; sulphur 290; chloride 61.

---

barium, chemical symbol Ba. Atomic weight 137.3. Has no use in the metabolism of animals or man, but in the form of its soluble salts is highly toxic. A fatal dose of barium chloride may be as low as 1g. Symptoms of poisoning include vomiting; colic; diarrhoea; slow irregular pulse; high blood pressure; convulsive tremors; muscular paralysis.

Has been used in female contraceptive devices but these were regarded as presenting a potential cervical cancer risk in susceptible individuals. Still used in the form of insoluble barium sulphate in 'barium meals', where it shows up the gastrointestinal tract on X-rays for investigational purposes.

---

barley, a low sodium food and a useful provider of potassium, phosphorus, iron, copper, zinc and sulphur. Boiling reduces levels of all minerals about threefold, mainly because of dilution and swelling with water. Minerals present are (in mg per 100g), for raw pearl barley and the boiled variety respectively: sodium 3, 1; potassium 120, 40; calcium 10, 3; magnesium 20, 7; phosphorus 210, 70; iron 0.7, 0.2; copper 0.12, 0.04;

zinc 2.0, 0.7; sulphur 110, 36; chloride 110, 36.

Basedow's disease,   *see* hyperthyroidism.

---

beansprouts,   useful source of iron and potassium but sodium content is introduced during canning. Minerals present in canned variety (in mg per 100g) are: sodium 80; potassium 36; calcium 13; magnesium 10; phosphorus 20; iron 1.0; copper 0.09; zinc 0.8; chloride 120.

---

beef,   excellent source of iron, zinc and sulphur with useful quantities of potassium, copper and sulphur. Sodium content reflects salt added during cooking and processing. All cuts when cooked contain minerals (in mg per 100g) in the ranges of: sodium 50-1000; potassium 160-400; calcium 6-18; magnesium 11-26; phosphorus 90-240; iron 1.4-3.5; copper 0.13-0.27; zinc 1.4-8.7; sulphur 220-310; chloride 51-1560.

---

beef extract,   very high sodium content because of salt addition but potassium also very high because of concentration of extract from original beef. Rich in iron, zinc, copper and phosphorus with useful quantities of calcium and magnesium. Mineral contents (in mg per 100g) are: sodium 4800; potassium 1200; calcium 40; magnesium 61; phosphorus 590; iron 14.0; copper 0.45; zinc 1.8; chloride 6800.

---

beer,   can supply useful potassium and iron intakes depending upon type, but is generally low in sodium and other minerals. In beers and lagers of all kinds, bottled or draught, quantities of minerals (in mg per 100g) are in the ranges of: sodium 2-23; potassium 33-130; calcium 3-14; magnesium 3-20; phosphorus 3-40; iron 0.01-1.21; copper 0.01-0.08; zinc 0.01-0.04; chloride 4-57.

---

beetroot,   low sodium food (except when salt is added during boiling) and an excellent provider of potassium with useful quantities of the other minerals. There is little difference in the mineral content between raw or boiled (in mg per 100g): sodium 64; potassium 350; calcium 30; magnesium

17; phosphorus 36; iron 0.4; copper 0.08; zinc 0.4; sulphur 22; chloride 76.

bentonite, a food additive that is a colloidal clay composed chiefly of hydrated aluminium silicate. Used as an anti-caking agent; clarifying agent. Acceptable daily intake not yet allocated. Permitted in certain wines and as a miscellaneous additive.

bilberries, virtually sodium free with some potassium and iron but only low potencies of other minerals. As raw contains (in mg per 100g): sodium 1; potassium 65; calcium 10; magnesium 2; phosphorus 9; iron 0.7; copper 0.11; zinc 0.1; chloride 5.

bioavailability, a measure of how much of a dietary mineral actually becomes available for utilization by the body. Depends upon the form in which the mineral is presented in the food; other factors in the food; how easily it is absorbed and assimilated; the body status of that particular mineral; ease of excretion. Examples of bioavailability of iron: 95 per cent is available from steak and corned beef; 75 per cent is available from bran cereal; 57 per cent from white bread; 10 per cent from a boiled egg. The low figure for eggs is due to binding of the iron by a specific protein in the food that becomes coagulated and resistant to digestion.

biscuits, good source of iron, calcium, phosphorus and zinc. High sodium because of added salt.
Homemade variety contains the following minerals (in mg per 100g): sodium 220; potassium 88; calcium 82; magnesium 12; phosphorus 84; iron 1.5; copper 0.11; zinc 0.5; chloride 340.
Shortbread variety contain (in mg per 100g): sodium 270; potassium 91; calcium 97; magnesium 13; phosphorus 75; iron 1.5; copper 0.12; zinc 0.5; chloride 440.

bismuth, chemical symbol Bi. Atomic weight 209. Not an essential mineral for animals or man but it has found widespread use in the past in the treatment of syphilis and yaws. Its insoluble salts are still used as protective agents in the gastrointestinal tract and by application to the skin.

Acute toxic effects include gastrointestinal disturbance; loss of appetite; headache; malaise; skin reactions; discoloration of mucous membranes; mild jaundice; blue line on the gums. Kidney changes may occur.

Chronic toxic effects include a nerve syndrome characterized by deterioration of mental ability, confusion, tremor, impaired co-ordination. Noticed mainly in colostomy and ileostomy patients taking insoluble bismuth subgallate over prolonged periods.

Medical uses of bismuth include:
1. treatment of syphilis by injection of the element or its salts;
2. antacid action in treating indigestion;
3. an astringent action in treating diarrhoea;
4. a protective action on mucous membranes and raw surfaces in those who have undergone colostomy or ileostomy.

---

bismuth carbonate, provides 80-82.5mg bismuth in each 100mg. Dose is 0.6-2g to a maximum daily dose of 15g. Used internally as a mild antacid in treating dyspepsia and gastric and duodenal ulcers. Used externally in mild irritant skin conditions. For toxic effects *see* bismuth.

---

bismuth subgallate, provides 46-52mg bismuth in each 100mg. Dose is 0.6-2g when used orally for its astringent properties in the treatment of diarrhoea, dysentery and ulcerative colitis. Administered by mouth to help control the odour and consistency of stools in those with colostomy or ileostomy.

Employed as a dusting powder for treating eczema and similar skin diseases. Incorporated into suppositories in the treatment of haemorrhoids. For toxic effects *see* bismuth.

---

blackberries, virtually sodium free with good quantities of potassium, calcium and magnesium. Useful source of iron. For raw and stewed fruit respectively (with or without sugar), minerals present (in mg per 100g) are: sodium 4, 3; potassium 210, 180; calcium 63, 54; magnesium 30, 26; phosphorus 24, 21; iron 0.9, 0.8; copper 0.12, 0.10; sulphur 9, 8; chloride 22, 19.

---

blackcurrants, good source of potassium, calcium, phosphorus and iron. Virtually sodium free. Mineral contents are reduced by stewing. With and without sugar (in mg per 100g), minerals contained are, for raw and stewed fruit respectively: sodium 3, 3; potassium 370, 320; calcium 60, 51; magnesium 17, 16; phosphorus 43, 37; iron 1.3, 1.1; copper 0.14, 0.12; sulphur 33, 28; chloride 15, 13.

body content, the minerals calculated to be present in a person of 70kg (155 pounds; 11 stone) weight are shown in Table 1. These figures are only average and in no way refer to a 'normal' value. Such a term is meaningless as healthy individuals may vary in their mineral content yet show no abnormality. Mineral levels may be affected by ageing because toxic trace minerals especially accumulate in the body as it gets older; by past and current medical history; by sex; by family and religious dietary trends; by local environment which can contribute varying quantities of minerals from air, water and food; by the presence of other minerals with an antagonistic effect against the desirable ones; by the time of day the body sample is taken (e.g. before or after meals); by the analytical techniques used to measure minerals.

Table 1: Minerals present in a person weighing 70kg (155 pounds; 11 stone)

Metallic minerals	grams	Non-metallic minerals	grams
calcium	1200	oxygen	43500
potassium	250	carbon	12590
sodium	70	hydrogen	6580
magnesium	42	nitrogen	1815
iron	6	phosphorus	680
zinc	2.3	chlorine	115
copper	0.072	sulphur	100
vanadium	0.025	silicon	18
tin	0.017	fluorine	2.6
manganese	0.012	iodine	0.013
molybdenum	0.008		
chromium	0.002		
nickel	0.002		
cobalt	0.001		

body odour,   due to over-activity of the sweat glands; to hormonal changes in the female; to metabolic upset, e.g. sweet smell (due to acetone) of the diabetic's skin and nitrogenous smells in the person suffering from kidney failure; to excess dietary intake of garlic. Many respond to skin application of powders containing zinc oxide or talc which absorb the substances producing the body odour; some respond to topical application of deodorants of other types. Oral treatment that is most effective includes a combination of magnesium (400mg), zinc (20mg), vitamin B_6 (25mg) and para-aminobenzoic acid (100mg) daily. These nutrients appear to act as waste scavengers, removing substances that give off acrid odours in the body.

boils,   a tender, inflamed area of the skin containing pus at the site of infection. Pus consists of dead, white blood cells, living and dead bacteria (usually Staphylococcus aureus) and fragments of dead tissue. Standard treatment is oral antibiotics. Studies have shown that people with recurrent boils had low levels of blood zinc. When they were supplemented with 25-50mg of the element daily, blood zinc levels rose and healing of the boils was accelerated. In addition, whilst blood zinc levels were maintained, new boils did not appear.

bone phosphate, edible,   a food additive that consists mainly of hydroxyapatite. Used as an anti-caking agent; as a mineral supplement. Provides 39.9mg calcium; 18.5mg phosphorus per 100mg. Acceptable daily intake up to 70mg phosphorus per kg body weight. A permitted miscellaneous additive.

bonemeal,   main constituent is calcium hydroxyapatite which provides 40mg calcium in 100mg plus 18.5mg phosphorus. Other constituents are protein, fat, amino sugars and traces of magnesium. Also available as amino-acid chelated bonemeal which provides 13.5mg calcium in 100mg, plus 7.5mg phosphorus. Usual daily dose of either is up to 6 tablets (i.e. 400-500mg calcium). Often used as an excipient or filler in tablet making.

borax,   also known as sodium borate; sodium tetraborate; sodium biborate; sodium pyroborate. Provides 11.9mg boron per 100mg borax.

boric acid, also known as boracic acid. Provides 17.5mg boron per 100mg boric acid.

---

boron, chemical symbol B. Atomic weight 10.8. Occurs in nature as various compounds at an abundance of 10mg per kg in the earth's crust.

Boron was shown to be an essential element for plants in 1910. There is no evidence that it is needed by animals and man. Human diets provide 2mg per day which is efficiently absorbed and excreted in the urine. Toxic symptoms appear at intakes of 100mg or so. For this reason, the FAO/WHO authorities have now banned boron (as boric acid) as a food additive and preservative. Boron, in daily intakes of 5-20mg, has been claimed to relieve the symptoms of arthritis, but the evidence is not very convincing.

Medicinal uses have included:

1. external application as a dusting powder or lotion (in the form of boric acid) to treat bacterial and fungal injections;

2. treatment of mouth ulcers, eye infections and as a nasal douche (in the form of a solution of borax).

Toxic effects of boric acid and borax include a red rash with 'weeping skin'; vomiting; diarrhoea — characterized by a blue-green colour; depressed blood circulation; profound shock; coma; convulsions. Fatal dose in adults is 15-20g; that in infants 3-6g. Repeated intakes of small amounts can lead to accumulative effects.

In children toxicity can occur by the application of boron-containing dusting powders to broken areas of skin. For this reason, such dusting powders should not contain more than 5 per cent boric acid or borax. Absorption from solutions applied to body cavities and mucous membranes can be significant, so such solutions are not recommended as douches for vagina, bladder, wounds and ulcers.

---

brain, rich in phosphorus, potassium, iron and zinc. Useful source of copper. High sodium content is due to salt added whilst boiling. Mineral levels, which vary slightly between boiled calf and lamb's brains, are (in mg per 100g): sodium 210; potassium 190; calcium 11-16; magnesium 15; phosphorus 320-380; iron 1.4-2.3; copper 0.23-0.42; zinc 1.4-1.5; chloride 200-250.

---

bran, low sodium food that supplies excellent intakes of all other minerals. Particularly rich in potassium, calcium, magnesium, iron, copper and zinc. In the wholewheat grain, most of the minerals are concentrated in the bran fraction. From wheat, minerals present (in mg per 100g) are: sodium 28; potassium 1160; calcium 110; magnesium 520; phosphorus 1200; iron 12.9; copper 1.34; zinc 16.2; sulphur 65; chloride 150.

Brazil nuts, practically sodium free with excellent quantities of potassium, calcium, magnesium, phosphorus, sulphur, iron, copper and zinc. Minerals present are (in mg per 100g): sodium 2; potassium 760; calcium 180; magnesium 410; phosphorus 590; iron 2.8; copper 1.10; zinc 4.2; sulphur 290; chloride 61.

bread, good source of potassium, calcium, magnesium, phosphorus, iron, copper, zinc and sulphur. High sodium and chloride is due to added salt during baking. Wholemeal bread is superior to white bread in all mineral content except calcium, which is added to white bread but not wholemeal.

Wholemeal bread provides quantities less than in wholemeal flour due to losses in baking and presence of extra water. Minerals present (in mg per 100g) are: sodium 540; potassium 220; calcium 23; magnesium 93; phosphorus 230; iron 2.5; copper 0.27; zinc 2.0; sulphur 81; chloride 860.

White (in mg per 100g): sodium 540; potassium 100; calcium 100; magnesium 26; phosphorus 97; iron 1.7; copper 0.15; zinc 0.8; sulphur 79; chloride 890.

brewer's yeast, fairly low in sodium but excellent provider of potassium, calcium, magnesium, manganese, iron, copper and phosphorus. Supplies significant quantities of chromium and selenium. Dried variety contains (in mg per 100g): sodium 121; potassium 1700; calcium 210; magnesium 231; manganese 0.53; iron 17.3; copper 3.32; phosphorus 1753.

broad beans, low sodium food (unless excess salt is added during cooking) that supplies good quantities of potassium, iron, copper and phosphorus. When boiled, minerals present (in mg per 100g) are: sodium 20; potassium 230; calcium 21; magnesium 28; phosphorus 99; iron 1.0;

copper 0.43; sulphur 27; chloride 14.

---

broccoli tops, low sodium food that is very good source of potassium, calcium, iron and zinc. Some magnesium, phosphorus and copper present. Mineral levels (in mg per 100g) for raw and boiled state respectively, are: sodium 12, 6; potassium 340, 220; calcium 100, 76; magnesium 18, 12; phosphorus 67, 60; iron 1.5, 1.0; copper 0.07, 0.08; zinc 0.6, 0.4; chloride 55, 37.

Brussels sprouts, almost sodium free, but very good source of potassium and zinc with all other minerals present. Quantities of minerals present (in mg per 100g) for raw and boiled respectively, are: sodium 4, 2; potassium 380, 240; calcium 32, 25; magnesium 19, 13; phosphorus 65, 51; iron 0.7, 0.5; copper 0.06, 0.05; zinc 0.5, 0.4; sulphur (figure for boiled only) 78; chloride 28, 16.

---

bruxism, grinding of the teeth, often carried on during sleep, that can give rise to dental problems. Has been overcome by increasing the dietary intakes of calcium (300-500mg daily) plus the B vitamin calcium pantothenate (100mg daily).

---

butter, a high sodium food because of salt added during production. Traces only of the other minerals. Salted, minerals present are (in mg per 100g): sodium 870; potassium 15; calcium 15; magnesium 2; phosphorus 24; iron 0.2; copper 0.03; zinc 0.15; sulphur 9; chloride 1340.

---

butter beans, a low sodium food that supplies significant quantities of potassium, magnesium, phosphorus, iron, zinc and sulphur. Mineral quantities present (in mg per 100g) are: sodium 16, potassium 400; calcium 19; magnesium 33; phosphorus 87; iron 1.7; copper 0.16; zinc 1.0; sulphur 47; chloride 2.

C

cadmium, chemical symbol Cd. Atomic weight 112.4. It is not an essential nutrient for man and can be toxic after high intakes. Occurs in nature associated with zinc ores, so it is liberated when zinc is extracted. Earth's abundance 0.1 to 0.2mg per kg.

At birth cadmium is absent from the body, but it is absorbed in very small amounts and accumulates over 50 years or so to a body content of 20 to 30mg. More than half of this is found in the liver and kidneys. At a concentration of 22.4mg per 100g it can damage the kidneys. Within the tissues and organs most cadmium is immobilized by complexing with a specific protein called metallothionein. This serves to detoxify cadmium and other toxic minerals by making them unavailable to the tissues and organs. When metallothionein is deficient or saturated, toxic effects of cadmium appear. Excretion is very slow at a level of only 0.01 per cent of body levels daily.

Sources of cadmium include the atmosphere in the vicinity of industrial smelting and plating plants; fertilizers such as superphosphates where 15-21mg per kg may be present; drinking water which can contribute 1.1 μg per litre (soft water provides more than hard since galvanized pipes contain cadmium), vegetables grown on land irrigated by contaminated water or polluted by factory waste; tobacco smoke, up to 5 μg per day, from which cadmium is better absorbed than from food and drink; dental amalgams.

Food sources of cadmium include oysters (3-4 μg per g wet weight); liver and kidneys (1-2 μg per 100g); fruits, vegetables and nuts (0.04-0.08 μg per g); soya beans (1 μg per g) that have been grown on soil heavily fertilized with salvage sludge. Muscle meats and milk are poor sources. Cadmium is lost by food refining and processing, as are the essential trace minerals.

Daily intakes of 55-70 μg per person have been proposed by WHO as tolerable. Calculated intakes have been reported as 60-90 μg per day for young adult female New Zealanders; from 27-64 μg per day in children confined to institutions; as 26 μg per day in daily food intakes of USA individuals; as ranging from 50-150 μg per day amongst various countries.

Competes with zinc, copper and selenium in absorption and metabolism probably by virtue of competition for some protein-binding sites.

Excessive intakes can cause anaemia, probably by antagonizing copper and iron functions in blood formation; high blood pressure, probably through kidney damage; injurious effects on the reproductive organs in animals; Itai-itai disease (see entry); atherosclerosis. Protection against excessive accumulation of cadmium is possible by adequate intakes of zinc, copper and selenium in the diet.

Acute toxicity effects after eating cadmium include nausea; vomiting abdominal cramps; shock; gastric and intestinal bleeding. After inhalation they are eye irritation; headache; vertigo; cough; constriction of the chest; weakness in the legs; difficulty in breathing; pneumonia.

Chronic toxic effects include yellow pigmentation of the teeth; soreness of the nostrils (cadmium sniffles); loss of smell; emphysema; pain in the back and limbs; bone changes leading to disability; loss of protein in the urine.

Medicinal forms of cadmium include:
1. cadmium sulphide, used in the control of seborrheic dermatitis and dandruff, usually in the form of shampoos. It may cause photosensitization.
2. cadmium salts, used as antihelmintics (to destroy parasitic worms) in swine and poultry.

---

calcitonin, also known as thyrocalcitonin. A peptide (chain of amino acids) hormone produced by specific cells of the thyroid gland. It is secreted in response to high blood calcium levels and its action is to reduce blood calcium by inhibiting the rate of calcium release from the bone. Used medically in the treatment of high blood calcium levels and in Paget's disease.

---

calcium, chemical symbol Ca. Atomic weight 40.08. An alkaline earth metal. Occurrence in the earth's crust is 3.64 per cent, the fifth most abundant element. Sea water contains 400g calcium per ton. Principal mineral in nature is limestone, also known as calcium carbonate, marble, chalk and dolomite.

Body content of calcium is about 1200g. At least 99 per cent of this is in the skeleton and teeth, mainly in the form of calcium phosphate. Total calcium outside the skeleton is no more than 10g. Much of this is in the nerves, muscles (including the heart) and the blood. Usual blood levels are between 8.5 and 10.5mg per 100ml; half is bound to plasma protein and the other half is ionic calcium. Ionic calcium is essential in the process of blood clotting. When ionic calcium is reduced — in deficiency or, for example, when blood pH becomes too alkaline, as after excessive vomiting — the nerves become over-susceptible to stimuli and twitching results. Clinically called tetany, the condition causes muscles to lose tone and become flaccid so that infants who lack ionic calcium are late in sitting, standing and walking.

Food sources of calcium include milk and cheese as the most valuable, but wholegrains, vegetables and pulses contribute meaningful amounts. Diets, for example, vegan, where cereals contribute a high proportion of energy will also supply most of the calcium. In hard-water areas, drinking water can supply a significant quantity of calcium, up to 200mg per day with an average of 75mg. Richest food sources are (in mg per 100g): hard cheese, 400-1200; soft cheese, 60-725; canned fish, up to 400; nuts, up to 250; pulses, up to 150; cow's milk, 120; root vegetables, up to 80; eggs, up to 60; oatmeal, up to 60; fruits, up to 60; wholewheat flour, up to 40. human milk, 3.5; maize, up to 18; fresh fish, up to 32. White flour has a higher content of calcium than wholewheat because it is fortified (usually with chalk) to give a level of 140mg per 100g. Unfortified white flour contains only half the level of calcium in wholewheat (or wholemeal).

Absorption of calcium is only between 20 and 30 per cent of that eaten. The body absorbs calcium more efficiently when low intakes are eaten and can adapt to prolonged or perpetual low levels in the diet. Children in Sri Lanka, India, South Africa (black) and Peru can subsist on 200mg daily; adults in Africa may receive only 300mg per day. In all these cases skeleton and blood maintain normal levels of calcium. Studies indicate that normal body levels are maintained by reduced excretion, suggesting more efficient absorption.

Normal subjects on Western diets need at least 600mg calcium daily in their diets to maintain positive balance, i.e. losses are less than intakes. Calcium absorption decreases with age, so the elderly need more in their diet to compensate. Hence in the population as a whole, the necessary daily intake is likely to be as high as 900mg per day to maintain balance.

Absorption is an active process requiring adequate oxygen and energy. Other food ingredients that assist in calcium absorption are:
1. vitamin D which is absolutely essential;
2. proteins which supply the amino acids needed to help carry calcium across the intestinal barrier;
3. lactose, the sugar present in milk, which must be digested first. Those who lack the lactose-digesting enzyme lactase may be more prone to calcium deficiency.

4. stomach acid, needed to dissolve calcium before absorption;
5. magnesium, which must be present in adequate quantity for calcium to be assimilated.

Food constituents that may prevent calcium absorption are:
1. phytic acid, present in raw cereals, raw vegetables and uncooked bran;
2. dietary fibre which contains uronic acid that can bind calcium;
3. phosphorus which in the form of phosphate can bind calcium when the phosphorus-calcium ratio in a food is very high, e.g. in junk foods. Ideal ratio is 1:1;
4. fats, particularly the saturated variety, which can form insoluble soaps with calcium;
5. Oxalic acid, which is present in high concentration in certain fruits and vegetables, e.g. rhubarb, can combine with calcium to form insoluble calcium oxalate that is not absorbed.

Excretion of calcium occurs in the urine, faeces and sweat. Between 100 and 350mg calcium is lost in the urine each day. Losses are higher in the summer. Night losses of urinary calcium increase after the menopause but losses may be reduced by milk drink before sleep. High-protein diets cause increased urinary loss of calcium; reduced protein intake gives rise to less urinary loss. When protein intake is high, increased absorption may be more than offset by increased urinary excretion.

Calcium in the faeces comes from two sources. At least 130mg per day comes from calcium secreted in the digestive juices of the intestine that are not reabsorbed. The remainder represents the unabsorbed fraction of dietary calcium. This varies depending on intake: when this is 600-1000mg, a normal adult absorbs less than half of it, so 400mg or more is lost in the faeces. With an intake of less than 500mg adaptive mechanisms increase the proportion absorbed. With severe calcium restriction (less than 200mg per day) the efficiency of absorption rises to 70-80 per cent, so less is excreted. The body absorbs calcium more efficiently by increasing its production of 1, 25-dihydroxy vitamin D_3, the active form of vitamin D_3, from the vitamin.

Losses in sweat are usually insignificant at about 15mg per day. Working in extreme heat can cause increased sweat losses up to 100mg per hour, which can contribute 30 per cent of total body losses of calcium, a significant figure if prolonged.

Metabolism of calcium in the foetus and growing child is geared to bone formation. In the human foetus the mineral is deposited at a steady rate from 12 weeks onwards but particularly rapidly from the 34th to 40th week when half the total birth calcium of 25g is laid down in the body. Over the last two to three months of pregnancy calcium is deposited in the foetus at a rate of between 200 and 300mg daily. The mother needs to increase her dietary intake accordingly. Once the child is born, it stills relies upon mother's milk to supply the essential calcium. Human breast milk yields some 250-300mg per day so this too must be accounted for in the diet of the nursing mother.

From birth to adolescence, as the bones develop, deposition of calcium varies from 60g during the first year of life to 90g per year as puberty approaches. The growing body must increase the percentage of calcium from around 0.8 per cent to 2.0 per cent during the development years. Hence utilization must be efficient and dietary intakes adequate.

Regulation of body calcium is under the control of vitamin D and the hormones calcitonin and parathyroid. The calcium in the blood and tissues forms a combined, interchangeable part of 4-7g. The concentration in blood plasma is kept within very narrow limits; absorption of dietary calcium and its excretion are also regulated with the aim of keeping skeletal stores constant. Control occurs at three sites: the intestines, the bones and the kidneys. Calcium in the bones is not static but is constantly being lost and replenished at the rate of 700mg per day. A slight fall in plasma calcium level stimulates secretion of parathyroid hormone from the parathyroid glands adjacent to the thyroid gland in the neck. The hormone increases calcium absorption from the small intestine and from the bone reserves. At the same time urinary excretion is reduced. Vitamin D, in its active form 1, 25-dihydroxycalciferol, also contributes to these effects. Once the plasma calcium rises, it has the effect of triggering the secretion of the hormone calcitonin from the thyroid gland, decreasing the secretion of parathyroid hormone, and the decline of production of 'active' vitamin D, 1 25-dihydroxycalciferol. The net result is reduced absorption of calcium from the intestine and inhibition of the cells that cause release of calcium from the bones (osteoclasts).

In the female, circulating oestrogens (sex hormones) reduce the sensitivity of bone to the calcium-mobilizing effects of parathyroid hormone. After the menopause, when oestrogenic levels decrease dramatically, bone calcium loss tends to increase at a greater rate than it can be replenished. The result is osteoporosis, a major cause of bone fractures in the elderly.

High-level thyroid hormone production can cause excessive loss of calcium from bone as can synthetic corticosteriods like prednisone and prednisolone.

Functions of calcium are:
1. building and maintaining healthy bones and teeth by the deposition

of hard crystals of calcium phosphate within a soft, fibrous organic matrix;

2. controlling the excitability of nerves and muscles;

3. maintaining the integrity of the cement substances that hold body cells together;

4. ensuring normal heart muscle function;

5. correct control of all muscle contractions;

6. normal conduction of nerve impulses;

7. controlled release of the hormones needed to induce lactation;

8. in the process of blood clotting;

9. in assisting intrinsic factor in the absorption of vitamin B_{12};

10. in controlling blood-cholesterol levels. In one trial, 1.5g of calcium was given orally at each mealtime to twenty patients over a period of four weeks. In each case blood-cholesterol and fat levels fell significantly. No effect was noted with injected calcium suggesting that oral calcium prevents cholesterol absorption from the diet.

Deficiency of calcium may be caused by:

1. low dietary intake in the food;

2. lack of vitamin D;

3. increased dietary intakes of phytic acid, uncooked bran, phosphate, animal fats, oxalic acid (see above);

4. hormone imbalance, i.e. too much calcitonin, thyroxine, corticosteroids, synthetic oestrogens as in the contraceptive pill or too little parathyroid hormone (see above);

5. malabsorption due to pancreatic insufficiency; coeliac disease; lactase deficiency; cow's milk allergy; rapid intestinal transit of food, reducing time available for absorption; complete lack of stomach acid (achlorhydria); reduced production of stomach acid (hypochlorhydria); diuretics, chronic intestinal infections and infestations;

6. repeated pregnancies without adequate intake;

7. prolonged breast-feeding with delayed weaning (in some communities up to 2 years);

8. kidney disease where urinary excretion of calcium is excessive but condition is rare.

Diseases and signs of calcium deficiency are:

1. rickets in children, characterized by excessive sweating of the head, restlessness, poor ability to sleep and constant head movements. Infants do not sit, crawl or walk early and closing of the soft joints in head bones is delayed. Weight-bearing as the infant grows eventually bends the bones, causing bow legs, knock-knees and pigeon breast. Rickets is more likely due to vitamin D deficiency but lack of calcium over long periods can also cause the disease;

2. osteomalacia in adults, characterized by bone pain, muscle weakness producing a characteristic gait and muscle spasms. Healing of fractures is delayed. Excessive outward curvature of the spine causing hunching of the back is common. Osteomalacia is usually due to vitamin D deficiency but calcium lack can give rise to similar symptoms:

3. osteoporosis, characterized by bone pain and ease of fracture of bones;

4. tetany, characterized by twitching and spasm of the muscles of the face, hands and feet.

Therapeutic uses of calcium are:

1. in treating rickets, osteomalacia, and the diseases of malabsorption, with 3.6g of calcium (in three doses) daily as one of the accepted calcium supplements;

2. in tetany where calcium gluconate may be injected intravenously for immediate relief or by oral administration of 3.6g calcium daily as one of the accepted supplements;

3. in osteoporosis at least 1g daily, preferably with vitamin D and sodium fluoride;

4. in cataracts, or preferably to prevent them, since prolonged low blood-calcium levels predispose to cataract formation;

5. in allergies of a gastrointestinal nature like coeliac disease, or those causing asthma, hay fever, eczema where lack of calcium can enhance histamine release, the cause of many allergies;

6. in those who are allergic to dairy products where elimination of these can give rise to lack of calcium and of vitamin D;

7. in those women who are post-menopausal and hence prone to osteoporosis;

8. in toxic metal exposure such as lead, mercury, aluminium and cadmium where high calcium supplementation can help eliminate the toxic mineral. *See* toxic minerals.

9. in treating depression, anxiety, panic attacks, insomnia and hyperactivity. Daily doses are usually between 1 and 2g calcium.

10. in treating joint and muscle pains and the arthritic condition. An extra 500-1000mg calcium required daily.

11. in ensuring the increased intake needed in pregnancy and whilst breast-feeding. Quantities vary, but an extra 700mg calcium daily will suffice.

12. used in relief of severe kidney, biliary or intestinal colic and the acute colic of lead poisoning when it is given intravenously;

13. used to reduce the toxic effects of excessive potassium in the blood which can lead to heart failure;

14. used to reduce the toxic effects of very high blood-magnesium levels.

Supplementary preparations of calcium are amino acid chelated calcium; bonemeal; calcium acetate; calcium ascorbate; calcium carbonate; calcium chloride; calcium glucobionate; calcium gluceptate; calcium gluconate; calcium glycerophosphate; calcium phosphate; calcium lactate; calcium laevulinate; calcium orotate; calcium sodium lactate; calcium tetrahydrogen phosphate; dibasic calcium phosphate; dolomite; tribasic calcium phosphate. *White flour* has chalk (calcium carbonate) added to it as a source of calcium.

Recommended daily intakes vary throughout the world, reflecting differing conclusions based on a variety of nutritional studies. May also reflect varying potein intakes and those of vitamin D provided by the diet and produced in the skin. UK and USA recommendations are respectively (in mg per day): 0-0.5 year, 600 and 360; 0.5-1 year, 600 and 540; 1-8 yrs, 600 and 800; 9-10 yrs, 700 and 800; 11-14 yrs, 700 and 800; 15-17 yrs, 600 and 1200; 18 yrs, 500 and 1200; 19 to 75+ yrs 500 and 800; during pregnancy 1200 and 1200; whilst breast-feeding 1200 and 1200.

WHO recommendations are 0-1 year, 500-600; 1-9 yrs, 400-500; 10-15 yrs, 600-700; 16-19 yrs, 500-600; during pregnancy and whilst breast-feeding 1000-1200mg. Some authorities believe in higher intakes than these since UK studies indicating that less than 600mg daily in the diet leads to negative balance and that high intakes will reduce chances of developing osteoporosis in later life.

Food additives that contain calcium are calcium aluminium silicate; calcium phytate; calcium hydrogen orthophosphate; calcium tetrahydrogen diorthophosphate; tricalcium diorthophosphate; dicalcium diphosphate; calcium hydrogen sulphite.

Excessive absorption of calcium gives rise to condition of hypercalcaemia - abnormally high blood levels of calcium. Calcium is supplied by over-absorption from the intestine or excess supply from the skeleton. In this state there may be deposition of the mineral in the kidneys, heart and other soft tissues of the body. In some infants and children, it is usually due to excessive intakes of vitamin D (usually as supplements), but others may develop the condition without any obvious cause. Symptoms are loss of appetite, vomiting, wasting, constipation, flabby muscles and characteristic facial appearance. Blood calcium, urea and cholesterol are often raised, as is the blood pressure. There may be mental retardation and brain damage. Fatality rate is high if not diagnosed early. Treatment is reduction of calcium and vitamin D intakes from all sources.

In adults hypercalcaemia results from excessive doses of vitamin D or increased production of parathyroid hormone. Also reported in patients with peptic ulcer and impaired kidney function who are treated with high milk diets and antacids. These conditions promote excessive calcium absorption. Treatment is either reducing vitamin D intake if excess vitamin D is the cause, or calcitonin if excess parathyroid hormone is the reason.

In healthy adults there is no danger of hypercalcaemia since controlling mechanisms of the body ensure the calcium from the food does not exceed that lost elsewhere. Excessive amounts are readily excreted.

Excessive quantities when given intravenously or in a kidney dialysis solution can cause cardiac arrest.

---

calcium acetate, provides 25mg calcium in 100mg. Used mainly as calcium source in solutions for kidney dialysis. Used as a food additive, E263. Functions as a sequestrant; to prevent mould growth; as a firming agent. No limit on acceptable daily intake. A permitted miscellaneous additive.

---

calcium alginate, a food additive also known as algin, E404. Functions as emulsifier; stabilizer; thickener; gelling agent. Acceptable daily intake up to 50mg per kg body weight. Permitted in certain cheeses; in reduced-sugar jam products.

---

calcium amino-acid chelate, provides 18mg calcium in 100mg. Claimed to be the most efficiently absorbed form of calcium because the mineral is chelated with amino acids. Usual supplementary dose is up to 6 tablets daily (500mg calcium).

---

calcium antagonists, also known as calcium blockers, are a group of drugs that appear to function by preventing or slowing the flow of calcium into muscle cells. These cells need calcium to activate contraction of heart and artery muscles. The regulation of calcium movement into heart muscle cells is thus critical to heart muscle tone, resistance and blood pressure. By blocking the flow of calcium by an antagonistic action, these drugs are valuable in treating angina pectoris, heart failure, high blood pressure, weak heart muscle, fast heartbeat and coronary artery spasm. Adverse effects of calcium antagonists include transient headache, flushing, lethargy, dizziness, allergic reactions, low blood pressure, palpitations and occasionally precipitation of anginal pain.

calcium ascorbate,   provides 10.3mg calcium in 100mg. Supplies both calcium and vitamin C (about 90mg). Originally used as source of ascorbic acid (vitamin C) but increasingly taken as calcium supplement since claims of better absorption of calcium. Used as a food additive, E302. Functions as an antioxidant; as a vitamin; in meat preservation. Acceptable daily intake not specified. Prohibited in raw and unprocessed meat.

calcium benzoate,   a food additive, E213. Functions as a preservative. Provides 11.9mg calcium per 100mg. Restricted to certain foods and quantity restricted.

calcium biphosphate,   known also as monobasic calcium phosphate, acid calcium phosphate, 'calcium superphosphate'. Provides 17.1mg calcium and 26.5mg phosphorus in 100mg. Chiefly used as calcium and phosphorus supplement in flour, foods and animal feeds. Used also as a food additive, E341. Functions as an improving agent; a buffer; a firming agent; an emulsifying salt; a sequestrant; a yeast food; an acid raising agent, a nutrient of calcium and phosphorus. Acceptable daily intake up to 565mg per kg body weight at normal calcium intakes. Permitted in certain cheeses; in reduced-sugar jam products; as an improving agent, as a miscellaneous additive.

calcium carbonate,   also known as chalk. Provides 40mg calcium in 100mg. Dissolves in stomach acid from which 20 per cent of a dose is absorbed. Prolonged high intakes can cause constipation, alkalosis and hypercalcaemia. Overdose usually arises when it is used as an antacid in treating stomach and duodenal ulcers. Used to fortify white flour with calcium. Used as food additive, E170. Functions as alkali; firming agent; release agent; dietary supplement. No limit on acceptable daily intake. Permitted in cocoa products; in jam and reduced-sugar jam; in certain wines, in bread; as a miscellaneous additive.

calcium chloride, provides 27.2mg calcium in 100mg. Hexahydrate provides only 18.3mg calcium in 100mg. Both forms used in intravenous injections at dose of 0.5-2g. Hexahydrate may also be given by mouth up to maximum dose of 8g daily. More gastric irritation than other oral calcium salts, so is well diluted with water.

Used as a food additive. Functions as a sequestrant; as a firming agent. No limit on acceptable daily intake. Permitted in some creams; in cheese; in dried-milk products; in condensed milk; in jam and reduced-sugar jam products; as miscellaneous additive.

---

calcium citrates, may be monocalcium citrate; dicalcium citrate; tricalcium citrate. All three are used as food additives, E333. Function as sequestrants; firming agents, buffers. Provide 9.5mg calcium per 100mg monocalcium citrate; 8.7mg calcium per 100mg dicalcium citrate; 8.0mg calcium per 100mg tricalcium citrate. No limit on acceptable daily intakes. All are permitted in certain cheeses; in jam and similar products; as a miscellaneous additive.

---

calcium dihydrogen di-L-glutamate, a food additive used as a salt substitute; as a flavour enhancer. Provides 12.0mg calcium per 100mg. Acceptable daily intake up to 120mg per kg body weight. Should not be given to infants under 12 weeks old. Permitted only in dietetic foods.

---

calcium di-sodium ethylene diamine tetra acetate, also known as calcium sodium EDTA; sodium calcium edetate. A food additive used as a sequestrant; a chelating substance. Provides 9.8mg calcium per 100mg. Acceptable daily intake up to 2.5mg per kg body weight. Permitted as miscellaneous additive restricted to canned fish, canned shellfish, glacé cherries.

---

calcium glubionate, provides 6.6.mg calcium in 100mg. Used in intramuscular and intravenous injections at dose of 90mg; child's dose is 18-45mg. By mouth dose is 0.3-3g daily, usually presented as a syrup containing 325mg calcium.

---

calcium gluceptate, also known as calcium hexahydroheptonate and calcium glucoheptonate. Provides 8.2mg calcium in 100mg. Injectable form of calcium usually preferred in treatment of hypocalcaemia tetany. Intramuscular dose is 36-90mg calcium; intravenous dose is 90-360mg calcium. Causes transient tingling sensation and chalk-like taste after intravenous administration.

---

calcium gluconate, provides 8.9mg calcium in 100mg. May be given as solution intravenously or intramuscularly at dose of 1-2g. Children's doses are: up to 1 year, up to 300mg; 1-5 yrs, 300-600mg; 6-12 yrs, 600-1000mg. Oral doses are 1-5g of gluconate (89-445mg calcium). Causes less gastric irritation than calcium chloride or calcium lactate and is tasteless, so is the preferred oral presentation. Used by injection to remove pain of lead poisoning and to detoxify. Injections should not be given to those on digitalis therapy.

Used as a food additive. Functions as a buffer; as a sequestrant; as a firming agent. No limits on acceptable daily intake. Permitted in jam and reduced-sugar jam products; as a miscellaneous additive.

---

calcium glycerophosphate, provides 19.1mg calcium in 100mg plus 14.7mg phosphorus. Usual daily dose is 200-600mg glycerophosphate, but up to 4000mg (equivalent to 764mg calcium) has been given. Mainly used in debilitated conditions and in convalescence, particularly in anorexia nervosa to gain weight. Alleged that glycerophosphate enables brain to assimilate phosphorus easier. Reported to be twice as effective as sodium fluoride in preventing dental caries and is much less toxic.

---

calcium heptonate, a food additive that functions as a firming agent; as a sequestrant. Provides 8.4mg calcium per 100mg. Permitted miscellaneous additive.

---

calcium hydrogen malate, a food additive used as a firming agent. Provides 13.1mg calcium per 100mg. Permitted in jams and similar products, as a miscellaneous additive.

THE DICTIONARY OF MINERALS | C

calcium hydrogen phosphate, also known as dibasic calcium phosphate, dicalcium orthophosphate and dicalcium phosphate. Provides 23.3mg calcium in 100mg plus 18mg phosphorus. Used as a source of both calcium and phosphorus at daily doses of 0.6-2g of phosphate; 1-5g in the USA. Has been used as a dietary supplement but main function is as a filler in tablet making. Used also as a food additive E341. Functions as an emulsifying salt; as a firming agent; as a yeast food; as a dietary supplement. Acceptable daily intake up to 330mg per kg body weight at normal calcium intakes. Permitted in some cheeses; as a miscellaneous additive.

calcium hydrogen sulphite, known also as calcium bisulphite. A food additive, E227 used as a preservative; a firming agent. Provides 19.8mg calcium and 31.7mg sulphur per 100mg. Acceptable daily intake 2.2mg per kg body weight. Permitted in most sugar products; in certain fruit juices; as a permitted preservative restricted to specified foods. Quantity restricted.

calcium hydroxide, a food additive used as a firming agent; as a neutralizing agent. Provides 54.1mg calcium per 100mg. Acceptable daily intake is not limited. Permitted in cheese; in certain cocoa products; as a miscellaneous additive.

calcium iodide, provides 43.2µg iodine in 100µg iodide. Used in a similar manner to potassium iodide. Daily dose is 60-300mg for clinical use. As a supplement 200-1200µg daily is sufficient. Toxicity as for potassium iodide.

calcium iodobehenate, provides 23.5µg iodine in 100µg iodobehenate. Used in a similar manner to potassium iodide. It is only slowly absorbed and is not irritant to the stomach. Daily dose is 500mg for clinical use. As a supplement 500-1500µg daily is sufficient.

calcium lactate, provides 13.0mg calcium in 100mg. Usual daily dose is 1-5g lactate (equivalent to 130-650mg calcium). Less irritant than calcium chloride and usually preferred as oral supplement and in therapy. Used also as a food additive E327. Functions as a buffer; as a firming agent. Acceptable daily intake is not limited. Permitted in jam and similar products; as a miscellaneous additive.

calcium laevulinate,　provides 13.1mg calcium in 100mg. Usual daily dose is 1g laevulinate daily (equivalent to 131mg calcium). Has been given orally, intramuscularly and intravenously and also as a suppository.

calcium malate,　a food additive used as a buffer; as a firming agent. Provides 23.3mg calcium per 100mg. Acceptable daily intake is not limited. Permitted in jam and similar products; with calcium carbonate in certain wines; as a miscellaneous additive.

calcium oxide,　a food additive used as an alkali; as a dietary supplement of calcium. Provides 71.4mg calcium per 100mg. Acceptable daily intake is not limited. Permitted in certain cocoa products (quantity restricted); as a miscellaneous additive.

calcium pectate,　a food additive, E440a. Functions as a stabilizer; as a gelling agent; as a thickener. Provides very small amounts of calcium per 100mg. Acceptable daily intake has not been specified. Permitted as an emulsifier; as a stabilizer; in certain jam products, quantity restricted.

calcium phosphate,　also known as tribasic calcium phosphate, tricalcium phosphate, calcium orthophosphate, and tricalcium diorthophosphate. Usual supplementary intake is 0.6-2g phosphate daily, but up to 5g is given as antacid. Although soluble in gastric acid, it becomes insoluble in the small intestine and is poorly absorbed. Often used as filler in tablets. Used also as food additive, E341. Functions as an anti-caking agent; as a buffer; as an emulsifying salt; as a dietary supplement; as a yeast food. Provides 38.7mg calcium and 18.7mg phosphorus per 100mg. Acceptable daily intake 374mg per kg body weight at normal calcium intakes. Permitted in some cheeses; in sweetened condensed milk containing added lactose; as a miscellaneous additive.

calcium phytate, a food additive that functions as a sequestrant. Provides 27.0mg calcium per 100mg. Permitted as a miscellaneous additive; in certain red wines.

---

calcium polyphosphates, food additives used as emulsifying salts. Permitted in certain cheeses; as a miscellaneous additive.

---

calcium propionate, a food additive, E282, used as a preservative; as an anti-fungal agent; as a 'rope' inhibitor in drinks. Provides 21.5mg calcium per 100mg. Acceptable daily intake is not limited. Permitted as a preservative; in bread, flour; confectionery; in Christmas puddings, quantity restricted.

---

calcium pyrophosphate, a food additive also known as diCalcium pyrophosphate; diCalcium diphosphate. Functions as a buffer; as a neutralizing agent; as a dietary supplement. Provides 31.5mg calcium and 24.4mg phosphorus per 100mg. Acceptable daily intake up to 70mg phosphorus per kg body weight at normal calcium intake. Permitted in certain cheeses; as a miscellaneous additive.

---

calcium saccharin, a food additive used as an artificial sweetener (500 times sweeter than sugar). Acceptable daily intake up to 2.5mg per kg body weight. Provides 8.6mg calcium per 100mg. Permitted in soft drinks; in reduced-sugar and diabetic jam products; as an artificial sweetener. Prohibited in ice-cream.

---

calcium silicate, a food additive used as an anti-caking agent. Provides 13.6mg calcium per 100mg. Acceptable daily intake is not limited. Permitted as a miscellaneous additive.

---

calcium soaps, also known as calcium salts of fatty acids. Usually confined to calcium stearate, calcium myristate and calcium palmitate. Food additives, E470, used as emulsifiers; stabilizers; anti-caking agents. Acceptable daily intake is not limited. Permitted to contain certain antioxidants; as emulsifiers or stabilizers; as additive to Dutch rusks (quantity restricted). Calcium stearate is a permitted miscellaneous additive.

calcium sodium lactate, provides 7.8mg calcium in 100mg. Usual daily dose is 0.3-2.0g sodium lactate (equivalent to 23.4-156mg calcium). Alleged to be more soluble and hence better absorbed than calcium lactate.

calcium sorbate, a food additive E262 used as fungicide; as a fungistat; Provides 15.3mg calcium per 100mg. Acceptable daily intake up to 25mg per kg body weight. Permitted preservative restricted to certain foods, quantity restricted.

calcium stearate, *see* calcium soaps. Provides 6.6mg calcium per 100mg.

calcium stearoyl-2-lactate, a food additive, E482, used as an emulsifier; as a stabilizer; as a whipping aid. Provides 4.5mg calcium per 100mg. Acceptable daily intake up to 20mg per kg body weight. Permitted to contain certain antioxidants; as an emulsifier and stabilizer; in bread, quantity restricted.

calcium sulphate, a food additive used as a firming agent; as a sequestrant; as a nutrient; as a yeast food. Provides 29.4mg calcium and 23.5mg sulphur per 100mg. Acceptable daily intake is not limited. Permitted as a miscellaneous additive.

calcium tartrate, a food additive used as a buffer. Provides 21.3mg calcium per 100mg. Permitted with calcium carbonate in certain wines.

calcium tetrahydrogen phosphate, provides 15.9mg calcium in 100mg plus 24.6mg phosphorus. Used to fortify white flour with calcium.

cancer, any malignant tumour that arises from the abnormal and uncontrolled division of cells that then invade and destroy the surrounding tissues. It is important that the diet of anyone suffering from cancer is adequate in all the essential minerals as part of the general approach to nutritional control of the complaint. However, one trace mineral of particular importance in the prevention and perhaps the treatment of cancer is selenium. Epidemiological evidence suggests that the population living in low selenium areas has a higher rate of cancer incidence than a comparable population living in a high selenium area. For example, in the United States where selenium intakes average 50-100µg per person per day the cancer rate is higher than in Bulgaria where the intake is about 250µg per person per day. Within the same country, those with higher blood selenium levels have a lower incidence of cancer than those with low blood selenium levels. Animal experiments have proved that some cancers can actually be cured with selenium supplementation. Selenium appears to function against cancer by:
1. stimulating the immune system that protects against cancer;
2. toughening the cell membrane and making it less prone to attack by cancer-producing antigens.
The quantity of selenium to act as a preventative is at least 200µg per day; for treatment more may be necessary to increase blood levels of selenium, perhaps up to 500µg per day. Daily intakes of 2000µg have been administered under medical supervision in the treatment of cancer without any detectable damage to the liver or other side-effects.

---

carrots, in the raw state provide good quantities of potassium, calcium, iron and zinc. All are reduced on boiling because of water uptake and losses into water. Canned variety is high in sodium because of added salt.

Old variety, raw and boiled respectively, contains (in mg per 100g): sodium 95, 50; potassium 220, 87; calcium 48, 37; magnesium 12, 6; phosphorus 22, 17; iron 0.6, 0.4; copper 0.08, 0.08; zinc 0.4, 0.3; sulphur 7, 5; chloride 69; 31.

Minerals present in young carrots (boiled and canned respectively, in mg per 100g) are: sodium 23, 280; potassium 240, 84; calcium 29, 27; magnesium 8, 5; phosphorus 30, 15; iron 0.4, 1.3; copper 0.08, 0.04; zinc 0.3, 0.3; sulphur (boiled variety only) 9; chloride 28, 450.

---

cashew nuts, a low sodium food that is an excellent source of potassium, magnesium, phosphorus and iron. Minerals present (in mg per 100g) are: sodium 15; potassium 464; calcium 38; magnesium 267; iron 3.8; phosphorus 373.

---

cauliflower, useful source of potassium, iron and zinc but boiled variety lower in all minerals because of water uptake and some losses into boiling water. Mineral contents (in mg per 100g), for both raw and boiled respectively are: sodium 8, 4; potassium 350, 180; calcium 21, 18; magnesium 14, 8; phosphorus 45, 32; iron 0.5, 0.4; copper 0.03, 0.3; chloride 31,14.

---

celeriac, a turnip-rooted variety of celery that is a low sodium food, providing very good intakes of potassium with useful quantities of calcium, iron and copper. When boiled, minerals present are (in mg per 100g): sodium 28; potassium 400; calcium 47; magnesium 12; phosphorus 71; iron 0.8; copper 0.13; sulphur 13; chloride 23.

---

celery, provides more potassium than sodium with small amounts of all other minerals. Most soluble minerals are reduced on boiling because of losses into boiling water. Quantities present in raw and boiled vegetable respectively (in mg per 100g) are: sodium 140, 67; potassium 280, 130; calcium 52, 52; magnesium 10, 9; phosphorus 32, 19; iron 0.6, 0.4; copper 0.11, 0.11; zinc 0.1, 0.1; sulphur 15, 8; chloride 180, 100.

---

cheese, all cheeses are high in sodium because of salt addition during manufacture. Very rich sources of calcium, sulphur and phosphorus; good sources of potassium, zinc and iron in the hard and processed varieties. Lower potencies in the soft varieties.

Camembert type (in mg per 100g): sodium 1410; potassium 110; calcium 380; magnesium 17; phosphorus 290; iron 0.76; copper 0.08; zinc 3.0; chloride 2320.

Cheddar type (in mg per 100g): sodium 610; potassium 120; calcium 800; magnesium 25; phosphorus 520; iron 0.40; copper 0.03; zinc 4.0; sulphur 230; chloride 1060.

Danish Blue type (in mg per 100g): sodium 1420; potassium 190; calcium 580; magnesium 20; phosphorus 430; iron 0.17; copper 0.09; chloride 2390.

Edam type (in mg per 100g): sodium 980; potassium 160; calcium 740; magnesium 28; phosphorus 520; iron 0.21; copper 0.03; zinc 4.0; chloride 1640.

Stilton type (in mg per 100g): sodium 1150; potassium 160; calcium 360; magnesium 27; phosphorus 300; iron 0.46; copper 0.03; sulphur 230.; chloride 1720.

Cottage cheese (in mg per 100g): sodium 450; potassium 54; calcium 60; magnesium 6.0; phosphorus 140; iron 0.10; copper 0.02; zinc 0.47; chloride 670.

Cream cheese (in mg per 100g): sodium 300; potassium 160; calcium 98; magnesium 10; phosphorus 100; iron 0.12; copper 0.04; zinc 0.48; chloride 480.

Processed cheese (in mg per 100g): sodium 1360; potassium 82; calcium 700; magnesium 24; phosphorus 490; iron 0.50; copper 0.50; zinc 3.2; chloride 1020.

Cheese spread (in mg per 100g): sodium 1170; potassium 150; calcium 510; magnesium 25; phosphorus 440; iron 0.69; copper 0.09; chloride 760.

---

chelation, from the Greek *chelos*, meaning claw; is the process whereby a mineral is incorporated into a ring structure by the chelating agent. The process is essentially transformation of an inorganic to an organically bound mineral. The resulting mineral chelate has a stability determined by the chelating group. There are three levels of stability:
1. strong chelates such as those formed by the chelating agents ethylenediamine tetra-acetic acid (EDTA) and D-penicillamine which are used in medicine to remove unwanted toxic minerals from the body. Once the chelate is formed it is strong enough to pass through the body unchanged and hence get excreted.
2. weak chelates such as mineral ascorbates, citrates, lactates and gluconates formed from the mineral and sugar-type residues have a stability comparable to mineral salts and are hence easily dissociated;
3. intermediate strength chelates can be either amino acid chelates or orotates. These are strong enough to be absorbed intact but weak enough for the mineral to be transferred to other groups within the body by normal metabolic processes. Amino acid chelates are true biological chelates since this is how the body absorbs certain minerals, stores them, transports them and utilizes them. Orotates are synthetic derivatives of the mineral with orotic acid and there is scant evidence of their functioning as such within the body.

Chelated minerals that occur naturally include iron in haemoglobin; iron in haemosiderin; iron in ferritin; magnesium in chlorophyll; zinc in insulin; manganese in transmanganin in the blood; copper in haemocyanin (found in the blood of insects, crabs, octopus); calcium in milk; chromium in yeast; selenium in yeast; cobalt in vitamin B_{12}.

---

cherries, low sodium food that supplies excellent amounts of potassium with small amounts of all other minerals. Little lost on stewing. For raw and stewed cherries respectively (in mg per 100g) minerals present are: sodium 3, 3; potassium 280, 250; calcium 16, 18; magnesium 10, 10; phosphorus 17, 17; iron 0.4, 0.3; copper 0.07, 0.08; zinc 0.1, 0.1; sulphur 7, 7; chloride, trace.

---

chestnuts, low sodium food with very rich potassium content. Useful quantities of calcium, magnesium, phosphorus and iron. The edible portion (in mg per 100g) contains the following minerals: sodium 11; potassium 500; calcium 46; magnesium 33; phosphorus 74; iron 0.9; copper 0.23; sulphur 29; chloride 15.

---

chick peas, sodium content increased dramatically on boiling because of added salt. Excellent supplier of potassium, calcium, magnesium, phosphorus, iron, copper and sulphur. Boiled variety has lower potencies of minerals because of water uptake. Bengal gram type (in mg per 100g), for raw and boiled respectively, contains: sodium 40, 850; potassium 800, 400; calcium 140, 64; magnesium 160, 67; phosphorus 300, 130; iron 6.4, 3.1; copper 0.76, 0.33; sulphur 180, 84; chloride 60, 1310.

---

chicken, main minerals supplied are potassium, phosphorus, iron, zinc and sulphur. Some calcium, magnesium and copper present, along with reasonable levels of sodium. When cooked, mineral contents are in the ranges (in mg per 100g): sodium 72-95; potassium 230-370; calcium 9-12; magnesium 20-27; phosphorus 160-220; iron 0.5-1.9; copper 0.11-0.25; zinc 0.7-3.1; sulphur 210-300; chloride 69-95.

---

chicory, supplies significant quantities of potassium only. In the raw state (in mg per 100g), it contains the following minerals: sodium 7; potassium 180; calcium 18; magnesium 13; phosphorus 21; iron 0.7; copper 0.14; zinc 0.2; sulphur 13; chloride 25.

---

chinese restaurant syndrome, also known as the Ho Man Kwok syndrome. Symptoms start 15 minutes after eating Chinese food and consist of a numbness at the back of the neck which gradually radiates to both arms and to the back. There is a general weakness and palpitation of the heart. Has been suggested that the monosodium glutamate which occurs naturally in soy sauce may provide a local high concentration of sodium that causes the unpleasant effects. Possibility also that the high glutamic acid content (an amino acid) may contribute to the reaction.

---

chloride, chemical symbol Cl. Atomic weight 35.5. Abundance in igneous rock is 0.031 per cent by weight; in sea water 1.9 per cent by weight, primarily as sodium chloride. An essential mineral form of chlorine in plants, animals and man.

Chloride is usually associated with sodium both in the food and in body fluids; high sodium levels are paralleled by high chloride levels and vice versa. In body fluids chloride is negatively charged (anion) and it neutralizes the positively-charged sodium and potassium (cations). Body content of chloride is about 115g. This amount is kept constant by excretion of excess in urine, sweat and the gastrointestinal tract. Most people are in positive chloride balance since intake on adequate diets is more than enough. In parallel with sodium, excessive losses can be caused by heavy sweating and by diarrhoea. In addition, chloride in the form of hydrochloric acid may be lost to a significant degree in persistent vomiting. Normal blood plasma levels of chloride lie between 348 and 376mg per 100ml.

Functions of chloride are:

1. to act as the main anion to sodium and potassium cations in maintenance of body water levels and neutrality;

2. to provide chloride for the production of hydrochloric acid by the stomach.

Food sources of chloride parallel these of sodium. Foods rich in sodium are rich in chloride; poor sources of sodium like fruits, vegetables, nuts and wholegrains are also poor providers of chloride. *See* sodium, and individual foods for contents.

Deficiency of chloride in body fluids is highly unlikely but may parallel excessive sodium losses. No symptoms can be attributed specifically to lack of chloride. The only possible local deficiency of body chloride is in the condition of achlorhydria where the stomach cells fail to produce hydrochloric acid. This is due to a breakdown in the production mechanism, not to lack of chloride.

Supplementary forms of chloride include: sodium chloride - 100mg provides 60.7mg chloride; potassium chloride - 100mg provides 47.6mg chloride. Hydrochloric acid may be taken as betaine hydrochloride; glutamic acid hydrochloride, or dilute hydrochloric acid. *See* hydrochloric acid.

Increased blood plasma levels of chloride are seen in anaemia; heart disease, kidney disease, pregnancy (eclampsia).

Decreased blood plasma levels of chloride are seen in diabetes; fevers; pneumonia.

Urinary excretion of chloride is increased in a diet rich in salt; rickets; liver cirrhosis. It is decreased in chronic kidney disease; early stages of pneumonia; cancer; gastritis.

Excessive dietary levels of chloride are likely only with increased salt and potassium chloride intakes. The toxic effects of both of these are related to the sodium and potassium moieties respectively (*see* sodium *and* potassium). No toxic effects have been attributed to chloride but it has been suggested recently that the high blood pressure-inducing effect of excessive salt intakes which may be mediated through the hormones renin and aldosterone could be a function of high chloride rather than high sodium in the diet.

---

chlorine dioxide, a food additive used as a bleaching and improving agent for flour. Acceptable level for flow treatment is up to 30mg per kg; from 30-75mg per kg for special purposes. Permitted only as a bleaching or improving agent.

---

chocolate, variable sodium content but not regarded as high. Good source of potassium and calcium but milk variety high in calcium because of milk added. Useful source of magnesium, phosphorus and particularly iron.

Milk variety provides (in mg per 100g): sodium 120; potassium 420; calcium 220; magnesium 55; phosphorus 240; iron 1.6; copper 0.30; zinc 0.2; chloride 270.

Plain variety contains (in mg per 100g): sodium 11; potassium 300; calcium 38; magnesium 100; phosphorus 140; iron 2.4; copper 0.70; zinc 0.2; chloride 100.

Filled variety contents (in mg per 100g) are in the region of: sodium 60; potassium 240; calcium 92; magnesium 51; phosphorus 120; iron 1.8; copper 0.45; chloride 180.

---

chromium, chemical symbol Cr. Atomic weight 52.0. Occurs in nature as chromite. Earth's crust contains between 100 and 300mg per kilogram. Exists in many forms but trivalent chromium is the only one that can be used by the body. An essential trace element for animals and man.

Total body content is adults in usually between 5.2 and 10.4mg but some communities contain more. Blood plasma concentrations should lie in the range 2.1-5.2μg per 100ml. Hair concentration ranges from 15.6-31.2μg per 100g. Low plasma and hair values are indicative of deficiency.

Body content of chromium in adults shows wide geographical variation. Europeans and North Americans have body levels less than 6mg; African natives have 7.45mg; those in the Middle East have 11.8mg; inhabitants of the Far East have the highest level of 12.5mg. Studies on post-mortem organs from North America indicated that 17.6 per cent of these contained no detectable chromium compared with only 1.6 per cent of tissues from residents of the Far and Middle East. There is a progressive decline in tissue contents in chromium as individuals age.

Skin contains a substantial part of the body chromium (2mg); bone contains 1.2mg; muscle 0.9mg and fat 0.3mg.

Absorption of chromium from the diet is poor. Only between 3 and 10 per cent is absorbed from food and this is in the organic form. When trivalent chromium is added to the food as the inorganic form only 1 per cent is absorbed. Chromium incorporated into growing yeast or presented as the amino acid chelate is much better absorbed at a figure between 10 and 25 per cent. Most chromium from the diet is excreted in the faeces but there is some loss through the kidneys, and urinary excretion ranges from 6-10μg.

Foods content of chromium varies widely. Rich sources are dried brewer's yeast, black pepper, liver, molasses, cheese, wheatgerm and wheat bran. Moderate amounts are found in beef, butter, oysters, shrimps, grain and cereal products. Poor sources include white flour, lobster, haddock, chicken, egg-white and skimmed milk. Torula yeast contains so little that it is used as a diet in the experimental induction of chromium deficiency in animals.

All refined foods are low or lacking in chromium. Wholegrains contain chromium in the bran and germ layers of the grain at a total concentration of 175µg per 100g. This is reduced to 23µg per 100g when wholegrain is refined to white flour. Brown rice loses 75 per cent of its chromium when polished and refined into white rice. Raw sugar loses 98 per cent of its chromium when converted into white sugar. Even peeling of vegetables removes a large proportion of the chromium content.

Chromium contents of food average (in µg per 100g): egg-yolk 183; molasses 121; dried brewer's yeast 117; beef 57; cheese56; calves' liver 55; grape juice 47; wholemeal bread 42; wheat bran 38; black pepper 35; raw sugar 35; chilli 30; rye bread 30; honey 29; old potatoes 27; apple peel 27; oysters 26; wheatgerm 23; new potatoes 21; margarine 18; chicken leg 18; spaghetti 15; cornflakes 14; butter 13; chicken breast 11; spinach 10; bananas 10; carrots 9; egg-white 8; haddock 7; oranges 5; green beans 4; mushrooms 4; strawberries 3; skimmed milk 2.

Alcoholic beverages are good sources of chromium; wines 45; beers 30; spirits 13.5.

Functions of chromium reside solely in its presence in glucose tolerance factor (GTF). No other functions of the mineral are known. GTF stimulates insulin activity directly by binding to both insulin itself and specific insulin receptors; inorganic chromium does not have this property. GTF appears to be an essential cofactor in the following functions:

1. it promotes glucose transport and uptake of it by the muscles and tissues;
2. it promotes glucose utilization in the synthesis of fats;
3. it stimulates oxidation of glucose;
4. it catalyses glycogen formation from glucose in liver and brain;
5. it increases the sensitivity of tissues to insulin;
6. it controls blood-cholesterol levels, keeping them at normal levels;
7. it reduces blood-fats levels;
8. it increases concentration of protective high-density lipoprotein (HDL);
9. it reduces incidence of arteriosclerotic plaques in the aortas of rats;
10. it stimulates amino acid transport and protein synthesis in skeletal muscle;
11. it stimulates synthesis of essential brain-nerve transmitters by enhancing the transport of the amino acids precursors across the blood brain barrier;
12. it controls some aspects of the immune response in disease resistance, including that of interferon against viruses;

13. it promotes glucose uptake by the 'satiety centre' in the brain, so helping to suppress hunger symptoms.

Deficiency of chromium:

1. gives rise to syndrome resembling diabetes in rats — giving chromium reversed the condition;

2. causes severe impairment of glucose tolerance characteristic of kwashiorkor and protein-calorie malnutrition in infants. In many the condition was rapidly and markedly improved by chromium treatment.

3. gives rise to diseases of the nerves even with normal insulin levels;

4. causes increased blood-cholesterol levels in aged male rats — giving chromium lowered blood cholesterol;

5. causes development of plaques in the aortas of rats;

6. gives rise to high blood-fat levels in rats;

7. induced increased blood-cholesterol levels in hospital in some patients;

8. is suggested by epidemiological studies to be a factor in heart disease;

9. occurs in alcoholism;

10. is a feature of hypoglycaemia.

Causes of deficiency include high intake of refined sugars and starches; a diet of highly refined and processed foods that have had the chromium removed; diabetes due to complete lack of insulin when excessive chromium is lost in the urine; prolonged slimming regimes; living in areas where chromium concentration is low in the soil; pregnancy; severe malnutrition in the developing countries; prolonged intravenous feeding; alcoholism.

Therapy with chromium has been successful in children and adults suffering from impaired glucose tolerance due to malnutrition; the diabetes of pregnancy; some cases of maturity-onset diabetes; reducing the high blood-cholesterol levels in some patients; some cases of hypoglycaemia.

Symptoms of deficiency include alcohol intolerance; nervousness; irritability; frustration; intolerance; mental confusion; weakness; depression; learning disabilities. With the exception of the first two, symptoms are similar to those found in hypoglycaemia. Early symptoms of diabetes, such as frequent passing of urine; thirst; hunger; weight loss; itching may be associated with chromium deficiency if this is the cause of the diabetic condition.

Supplementary forms are inorganic trivalent chromium salts, e.g. chromium chloride, chromium acetate; amino acid chelated chromium; yeast, which contains GTF, is the preferred one. GTF is approximately 50 times as effective as inorganic chromium and at least 20 times more readily absorbed. GTF from yeast is some 10 times as effective as the chromium in foods such as liver, wheatgerm, and seafoods.

Recommended dietary intake is suggested by the US Food and Nutrition Board, National Research Council - National Academy of Sciences (1980) as follows (in μg per day): infants 0-0.5 year, 10-40; 0.5-1 year, 20-60; children and adolescents 1-3 yrs, 20-80; 4-6 yrs, 30-120; 7-10 yrs, 50-200; 11+ yrs, 50-200; adults 50-200. These suggestions take no note of the absorption of different chromium sources. Whilst a diet containing 30μg or less of GTF may be adequate, several hundred μg of inorganic trivalent chromium may be required.

Toxicity of chromium is low because so little of it is absorbed. Cats can tolerate 1000mg per day of trivalent chromium salts; rats showed no adverse effects from 100mg per kg diet. Lifetime exposure to 5mg per litre of trivalent chromium in the drinking water induced no toxic effects in rats and mice. Exposure of mice for three generations to chromium oxide at levels up to 20mg per kg of the diet had no effect upon mortality, growth or fertility of the animals.

Chronic exposure to chromium dust (in the form of chromate) has been associated with increased incidence of lung cancer. Oral administration of 50mg of chromate per kg has been associated with growth depression and liver and kidney damage in experimental animals.

Hexavalent chromium is much more toxic than trivalent chromium, but the former is never used in therapy or in supplementation, nor does it occur in natural foods.

See also diabetes, glucose tolerance factor.

---

chromium trichloride, also known as chromic chloride. Provides 32.8μg chromium in 100μg chloride. Used as a chromium supplement in patients with impaired glucose tolerance. Daily dose is 460μg to provide 150μg chromium.

---

cider, main attribute is as good provider of potassium and iron. Minerals present (in mg per 100g) are: sodium 7; potassium 72; calcium 8; magnesium 3; phosphorus 3; iron 0.49; copper 0.04; chloride 6.

---

cobalt, chemical symbol Co. Atomic weight 58.9. Widely distributed in nature. Abundance in earth's crust 0.001-0.002 per cent. Occurs as cobaltite, linnaeite, smaltite, erythrite.

Essential trace mineral only as a constituent of vitamin B_{12}. Ruminants have a requirement only for cobalt as the micro-organisms in their rumens can incorporate the mineral into vitamin B_{12}. Other animals and man cannot do so and a dietary source of the vitamin is essential for health. Vitamin B_{12} can only be synthesized by micro-organisms.

Body content of cobalt averages 1.1mg. Forty-three per cent of this is stored throughout the muscle tissues; 14 per cent is in the bone; the remainder is mainly distributed throughout the other tissues but mainly in the liver and kidneys. Blood levels vary over a wide range, from 0.007-0.036µg cobalt per 100ml whole blood in one study and from 0.17-1.5µg cobalt in another. Most of the cobalt of blood is found in the red blood cells rather than in the plasma.

Dietary intakes of cobalt depend upon the amount of mineral in the soil and hence in the plants and animals that thrive on that soil. Children in the USA were found to have diets containing from 0.25-0.69mg cobalt per kg food. In diets of adults, intakes varied from 0.30-1.77mg cobalt per day. Much lower levels are found in the diets of most Japanese who eat only 0.01mg daily. WHO sources recommend a minimum daily intake of 1µg cobalt to be absorbed.

Food sources that are rich in cobalt include fresh, green, leafy vegetables and some fish; poor sources are cereal and dairy products. Typical values are (in µg per 100g): vegetables 20-60; scallops 225; cod 120; liver 15; kidney 25; muscle meats 12; dairy products 1-3. Some of the cobalt in meat, fish and dairy products is present in their vitamin B_{12} content and the rest is the mineral in some other form. In vegetables and cereals, all is present in some other form.

It has also been used to reduce high blood pressure because of its action in causing dilatation of blood vessels, but quantities of 50mg oral cobalt chloride daily were required for periods up to 65 days.

In animals high intakes (4-10mg cobalt per kg body weight) can cause anaemia, loss of appetite and low body weight.

Functions of cobalt reside only in its presence in vitamin B_{12}. Many of the vitamin's functions are mediated through the cobalt portion of the molecule and they include synthesis of DNA; production of red blood cells; synthesis of methionine; synthesis of choline; synthesis of creatine. All of these involve transfer of active methyl groups from folic acid (B vitamin) to cobalt and hence to receptor substance. Other functions include maintenance of myelin, the fatty sheath that insulates nerves, and detoxification of cyanide introduced through food and tobacco smoke.

Deficiency of mineral cobalt is unknown but deficiency of vitamin B_{12} causes pernicious anaemia. This anaemia cannot be treated with cobalt

— it responds only to injections of the vitamin.

Therapy with cobalt has been used in the past to try and stimulate the bone-marrow to produce more red and white blood cells, but there is no convincing evidence that it helps. *Therapeutic forms* include cobaltous carbonate; cobaltous chloride; cobaltous nitrate. These are usually added to animal feeds.

Food additives containing cobalt are no longer used. Once it was added during the beer-brewing operation to improve the quality of the 'head' of the glass. This practice led to toxicity effects (see below) and the practice is no longer carried out.

Toxic effects of cobalt are highly unlikely with intakes from a normal diet. When used therapeutically in doses of 29.5mg daily side-effects included goitre, hypothyroidism and heart failure. Intakes of up to 17.7mg daily by heavy beer drinkers who drank up to 12 litres of beer (cobalt content about 1.5mg per litre) caused heart disease and death. Protein intake in these people was low; high-protein dietary levels are believed to protect against cobalt toxicity. Other toxic effects of cobalt noted in animals and human beings include overproduction of red cells (polycythaemia vera).

---

cobaltous carbonate, provides 25.9mg cobalt in 100mg carbonate (as hexahydrate). A nutritional factor used in cobalt or vitamin B_{12} deficiency in ruminants.

---

cobaltous chloride, provides 24.7mg cobalt in 100mg chloride (as hexahydrate). A nutritional factor used in cobalt or vitamin B_{12} deficiency in ruminants. Large amounts may lead to death in children. Toxic effects include skin flushing; chest pains; dermatitis; tinnitus (ringing in the ears); nausea; vomiting; nerve deafness; myxoedema; heart failure.

---

cobaltous nitrate, provides 20.0mg cobalt in 100mg nitrate (as hexahydrate). A nutritional factor used in cobalt or vitamin B_{12} deficiency in ruminants. Has been used as a dietary supplement of cobalt in man.

---

cocoa, rich source of sodium but even richer in potassium. Excellent provider of all minerals. The powder supplies the following (in mg per 100g): sodium 950; potassium 1500; calcium 130; magnesium 520;

phosphorus 660; iron 10.5; copper 3.9; zinc 6.9; chloride 460.

coconut, should be regarded as a good provider of potassium, magnesium, phosphorus, iron, copper and zinc. A low sodium food, the desiccated variety is richer in all minerals than the fresh nut. Mineral contents are for fresh and desiccated respectively (in mg per 100g): sodium 17, 28; potassium 440; 750; calcium 13, 22; magnesium 52, 90; phosphorus 94, 160; iron 2.1, 3.6; copper 0.32, 0.55; zinc 0.5, (desiccated not measured); sulphur 44, 76; chloride 110, 220.

cod liver oil, contains the following minerals, in trace amounts only; sodium; potassium; calcium; magnesium; phosphorus; iron; copper; zinc; sulphur; chloride.

coffee, fairly low in sodium but very rich in potassium, calcium, magnesium, phosphorus, iron, copper and sulphur. As a drink, all concentrations are reduced. The instant variety is richer in all minerals than ground coffee because it is concentrated.

Ground, roasted variety (in mg per 100g): sodium 74, potassium 2020; calcium 130; magnesium 240, phosphorus 160; iron 4.1; copper 0.82; sulphur 110; chloride 24.

Infused ground coffee (in mg per 100g): sodium trace; potassium 66; calcium 2; magnesium 6; phosphorus 2; iron trace; copper trace; chloride trace.

Instant variety (in mg per 100g): sodium 41; potassium 4000; calcium 160; magnesium 390; phosphorus 350; iron 4.4; copper 0.05; zinc 0.5; chloride 50.

coffee and chicory essence, rich source of potassium with useful quantities of all other minerals. Quantities present (in mg per 100g) are: sodium 65; potassium 750; calcium 30; magnesium 39; phosphorus 90; iron 0.7; copper 0.6; chloride 85.

cold, viral infection of the upper respiratory tract. Also know as coryza, rhinitis, cold in the head.

Symptoms have been relieved by sucking lozenges containing 23mg zinc, as a zinc gluconate, per lozenge every two wakeful hours. In the trial, 20 per cent of those with colds for less than three days lost their cold symptoms within 24 hours; none sucking a placebo lozenge did. After a week, 86 per cent of those with colds who had taken zinc recovered; half of those taking placebo lozenges still had symptoms. Zinc tablets that are swallowed do not have any beneficial effect in relieving cold symptoms so it is possible that the mineral has a direct action on the cold viruses in the mouth, nose and throat which stops their multiplication.

---

cold sores, caused by a herpes virus. They begin as small tender lumps on the lips, tongue, roof of the mouth, gums or cheek, usually preceded by a tingling or itching sensation. Lumps usually develop into painful ulcerations that form a scab in about a week. Healing takes between ten days and three weeks. Cold sores may be prevented or treated with supplementary zinc. Studies indicate that 25-50mg of elemental zinc daily is needed for therapy. Complementary vitamin C (500mg daily) may also help. Zinc creams applied directly to a developed cold sore have been claimed to accelerate healing. The mineral apparently blocks reproduction of the virus, allowing natural healing to proceed. *See also* cold.

---

compound cooking fat, trace amounts only of the following minerals (in mg per 100g): sodium, potassium, calcium; magnesium; phosphorus; iron; copper; zinc; sulphur; chloride.

---

confectionery, depending on type can supply good quantities of potassium, calcium, magnesium, iron and copper. Most are fairly low in sodium, but toffees of all sorts are high in sodium because of added salt.
Boiled sweets (in mg per 100g): sodium 25; potassium 8; calcium 5; magnesium 2; phosphorus 12; iron 0.4; copper 0.09 chloride 68.
Fruit gums (in mg per 100g): sodium 64; potassium 360; calcium 360; magnesium 110; phosphorus 4; iron 4.2; copper 1.43; chloride 160.
Liquorice allsorts (in mg per 100g): sodium 75; potassium 220; calcium 63; magnesium 38; phosphorus 29; iron 8.1; copper 0.39; chloride 120.
Pastilles (in mg per 100g): sodium 77; potassium 40; calcium 40; magnesium 12; phosphorus trace; iron 1.4; copper 0.32; chloride 120.
Peppermints (in mg per 100g): sodium 9; potassium trace; calcium 7;

magnesium 3; phosphorus trace; iron 0.2; copper 0.04; chloride 22.

Toffees, mixed (in mg per 100g): sodium 320; potassium 210; calcium 95; magnesium 25; phosphorus 64; iron 1.5; copper 0.40; chloride 480.

cooking losses, minerals cannot be destroyed but they are leached from food during cooking processes. Losses can be recovered completely by utilizing the cooking water. More minerals are lost from food boiled in soft water than in the hard variety. Losses of some minerals can be significant and are shown in Table 2. The figures are taken from a variety of sources and the degree of hardness of the water was not always mentioned. Losses into water are increased by using larger volumes of water and by pressure cooking which increases the temperature. If the water is used for gravy, sauces etc., all minerals can be recovered. Soaking in cold water overnight may also cause losses of some minerals in vegetables.

Table 2: Percentage loss of elements from vegetables after boiling

	Chromium	Cobalt	Copper	Magnesium	Manganese
Broccoli	44	63	93	53	70
Carrots	18	94	29	42	40
Endive	23	60	38	70	50
Green beans	40	49	87	58	49
Kidney beans	19	71	22	58	45
Peas	41	82	37	49	54
Potatoes	38	71	26	38	96
Spinach	42	60	64	61	75

copper, chemical symbol Cu, from the Latin *cuprum*. Atomic weight 63.5. Occurrence in earth's crust is 70mg per kg; in sea water present at a concentration of 0.001-0.02mg per litre. Naturally-occurring minerals are native copper, chalcocite, bornite, tetrahedrite; enargite, antlerite. An essential trace element for man, animals and many plants.

Body content of copper in adults ranges from 75-150mg. Low concentrates are present in the glands, bone and muscle, but because of their large mass the skeleton and muscles contain some 50 per cent of body copper. The liver is a rich source with about 10 per cent of total body copper contained in it. Brain, heart and kidney contain significant amounts. As an adult ages, liver copper content decreases but that of brain increases until the concentration in both is similar. The significance of this is not known.

The liver of a new-born baby contains between five and ten times the concentration of copper present in an adult liver. In the later months of pregnancy copper is transferred from the mother's liver to that of the foetus. This reserve is essential for the first few months of the new-born baby's life, since milk is not a good source of the mineral. Prematurely-born babies who do not get the chance of building up reserves of copper are more prone to deficiency in the first months of life than are those who are full term.

Blood plasma contains 90 per cent of blood copper in association with ceruloplasmin, an alpha-2-globulin with some bound loosely to plasma albumen. The red blood cells contain the remaining 10 per cent. Serum levels are usually between 100 and 200µg per 100ml. The protein complex in blood is very stable and this means that very little copper is excreted in the urine. Plasma copper rises during pregnancy and whilst being treated with oestrogens.

Excretion of copper is mainly in the faeces. It is transferred from the blood to the liver where it is stored and controlled. About 80 per cent of the copper absorbed into the liver is incorporated into the bile from where it is secreted into the intestine and hence disposed of in the faeces.

Food content of copper is widespread but its concentration is varied. The riches sources are (in mg per 100g): liver 2.5-11.0; oysters 7.6; whelks 7.2; crab 4.8; dried brewer's yeast 3.32; olives 1.60; hazel nuts 1.35; shrimps 0.80; dried lentils 0.76; oat flakes 0.74; rye bread 0.66; cod 0.55; poultry 0.2-0.3; wholemeal bread 0.27; peanuts 0.27; peas 0.23; dried fruit 0.2-0.4; potatoes 0.16; fresh fruits 0.1-0.2.

Non-food sources of copper include that added during the processing and storage of food; many pesticides and fungicides contain copper and some may be retained in foods; liquids that have been stored or processed in copper containers; copper pipes used to carry drinking water - if this is soft more copper will dissolve in it; water boiled in copper kettles where the protective chrome has been rubbed off; hot water from copper-lined heaters. Corrosion of copper pipes with soft water can contribute 1.4mg copper per day to the intake; that from hard water will provide less than 0.5mg copper per day.

Medicinal sources of copper include copper sulphate used in expectorants, cough suppressants, mucolytics and decongestants; at a concentration of 1mg per litre to prevent the growth of algae in swimming pools, reservoirs and ponds; at a concentration of 6mg per litre to kill fresh-water snails. Copper chloride, copper acetate and copper subacetate are used in the same manner as copper sulphate.

Functions of copper are:

1. as cofactor for many enzymes including that needed for the formation of melanin, the pigment that confers colour to hair and skin; those needed for connective tissue formation such as collagen and elastin, e.g. lipyl oxidase; those that are concerned with protection of body cells from oxidizing and other toxic agents, e.g. superoxide dismutase; those concerned with the transfer of oxygen, e.g. cytochrome oxidases; those concerned with nerve-impulse transmission in the brain, e.g. dopamine hydroxylase;
2. in blood formation where it is needed for iron transfer from ferritin and incorporation into haemoglobin;
3. in the absorption of iron from the food;
4. in the formation of healthy bone;
5; in developing resistance to illness through the white blood cells.

Deficiency in animals grazing on land deficient in the mineral gives rise to anaemia in cattle; osteoporosis in sheep; swayback (ataxia) in sheep characterized by shaky movements and unsteady gait.

Deficiency in human beings has been noted in:

1. malnourished children who live on diets deficient in protein and calories;
2. children unable to absorb nutrients because of malabsorption diseases like sprue;
3. infants with anaemia associated with depressed serum iron;
4. premature babies whose liver reserves of copper have not been built up;
5. hospital patients being fed intravenously or on kidney dialysis where the appropriate feed fluids lack copper;
6. children born with genetic defect that prevents normal absorption of copper (*See* Menke's syndrome);
7. those treated with chelating agents to remove toxic minerals from the body — the agents may also remove copper;
8. those living exclusively on highly refined diets devoid of copper;
9. those who lack the ability to absorb copper;
10. children who suffer from prolonged diarrhoea;
11. those who have excessive amounts of zinc, cadmium, fluorine or molybdenum in their diets;
12. those who have excessive intakes of phytic acid in their diets which can immobilize copper as insoluble copper phytate.

Deficiency symptoms in babies are failure to thrive; pale skin; diarrhoea; depigmentation of hair and skin; prominent dilated veins in the skin.

Deficiency symptoms in adults are anaemia, where it occurs after prolonged intravenous feeding following extensive bowel surgery; retarded growth; water retention; nervous irritability; brittleness of bones due to osteoporosis; chronic or recurrent diarrhoea; hair depigmentation; poor hair texture; low white blood-cell count that leads to decreased resistance to illness; loss in the sense of taste.

Therapy of deficiency is usually with copper sulphate but copper gluconate and amino acid chelated copper may also be used. Usual dose is up to 5mg elemental copper taken as required. These copper preparations are also used in supplementation where up to 2mg per day copper is usually sufficient.

Food additives that contain copper are copper chlorophyll; copper chlorophyllins: these are complexes of the mineral with chlorophyll where copper replaces magnesium. They are permitted colours.

Recommended daily intakes are suggested only by the US Food and Nutrition, National Research Council — National Academy of Sciences (1980). They are (in mg per day): infants 0-0.5 year, 0.5-0.7 year; 0.5-1.0 year, 0.7-1.0; 1-3 yrs, 1.0-1.5; 4-6 yrs, 1.5-2.0; 7-10 yrs, 2.0-2.5; 11 + yrs, 2.0-3.0; adults, 2.0-3.0.

High blood levels of copper are seen in those taking the contraceptive pill; in epilepsy; in zinc deficiency; in those with high blood cholesterol; in schizophrenia; in rheumatoid arthritis. High heart levels are seen in those dying of heart attacks. Nutrients that reduce high copper levels are vitamin C; zinc; manganese; rutin, which chelates copper before removal as a complex.

Therapeutic uses of copper are in treating anaemia that is due to copper deficiency (rare); in treating rheumatoid arthritis (*see* copper bangles); in IUD contraception (*see* intra-uterine devices); treating any deficiency condition mentioned above.

Toxicity of copper is generally low. Excess may result from hereditary disorders of copper metabolism (*see* Wilson's disease *and* Indian childhood cirrhosis); excessive intake of copper orally; addition of too much copper to or accidental contamination of intravenous feeding solutions or kidney dialysis solutions.

Manifestations of acute high concentration copper intoxication include nausea, vomiting, abdominal pain, diarrhoea, diffuse muscle pains. Eventually abnormal mental states develop, leading to coma and death due to metabolic acidosis and pancreatitis. Extensive haemolysis (bursting) of red blood cells leads to anaemia.

Dietary treatment of copper excess is a mixture of zinc and manganese in the ratio 20:1 which increases copper excretion via the urine.

copper bangles, traditional preventative and curative therapy for arthritis when worn on the wrist or ankle. Generally believed that copper dissolves in the acid secretion of skin and is then absorbed in a form that can be utilized in the body. Blood levels of copper in arthritis are usually high but mineral is in a non-utilizable form. Confirmation that this hypothesis is true has came from studies indicating that fat-soluble copper salicylate (aspirin) complexes are absorbed through the skin. They are strikingly effective in reducing the inflammation of artificially-induced arthritis in animals and of the clinical condition in man.

copper chlorophyll, a food additive used as a colouring agent, E141. Also designated Colour Index No. 75810, Natural Green 3. Acceptable daily intake up to 15mg per kg body weight. Permitted in certain jam products; in specified sugar products; in certain cheeses; as a colouring agent. May also be referred to as copper chlorophyllins.

copper sulphate, in the crude form is known as blue copperas; blue stone; blue vitriol. Provides 25.4mg copper in 100mg sulphate. Supplementary oral intakes are up to 10mg sulphate daily. At a strength of 1mg per ml a solution has been used as an antidote in phosphorus poisoning. A solution containing 10mg per ml has been applied to the skin to treat phosphorus burns. Solutions containing up to 1mg per litre water are used to prevent algae growth in ponds, swimming pools and reservoirs; at 5mg per litre it is used to kill disease-carrying fresh-water snails.

Large oral quantities of copper sulphate cause nausea; vomiting; metallic taste; burning sensation in the oesophagus and stomach. Later convulsions, low blood pressure and coma occur with kidney damage and liver damage. Doses of 1g have caused death.

cornflour, main attribute is a good content of iron. Quantities of minerals present (in mg per 100g) are: sodium 52; potassium 61; calcium 15; magnesium 7; phosphorus 39; iron 1.4; copper 0.13; zinc trace; sulphur 1; chloride 71.

cranberries, low sodium food that is rich in potassium and iron. Traces only of other minerals. Minerals levels for raw fruit (in mg per 100g) are: sodium 2; potassium 120; calcium 15; magnesium 8; phosphorus 11; iron 1.1; copper 0.14; sulphur 11; chloride trace.

cream, a low sodium food supplying good quantities of calcium, phosphorus and potassium with useful amounts of the trace minerals.

Single cream provides (in mg per 100g): sodium 42; potassium 120; calcium 79; magnesium 6; phosphorus 44; iron 0.31; copper 0.20; zinc 0.26; chloride 72.

Double cream provides (in mg per 100g): sodium 27: potassium 79; calcium 50; magnesium 4; phosphorus 21; iron 0.20; copper 0.13; zinc 0.17; chloride 46.

Whipping variety provides (in mg per 100g): sodium 34; potassium 100; calcium 63; magnesium 5; phosphorus 27; iron 0.25; copper 0.16; zinc 0.21; chloride 58.

Sterilized, canned variety (in mg per 100g): sodium 56; potassium 120; calcium 80; magnesium 6; phosphorus 44; iron 0.30; copper 0.20; zinc 0.26; chloride 140.

cream of magnesia, an aqueous suspension of hydrated magnesium oxide containing the equivalent of 7.45-8.35 per cent of magnesium hydroxide. Ten ml contains the equivalent of 550mg of magnesium oxide providing 300mg magnesium.

cretinism, also known as congenital hypothyroidism, juvenile hypothyroidism; a syndrome of dwarfism, mental retardation and coarseness of the skin due to lack of thyroid hormone from birth. May affect as many as 20 per cent of the population in isolated areas of Nepal, the Andes, Zaire and New Guinea. Iodine deficiency during foetal or early life may lead to cretinism in the child.

Cretins are often associated with particular areas where iodine is deficient in the soil and water supply. Infants afflicted have a characteristic look: the tongue is enlarged, lips are thickened, mouth stays open and drooling. Face is usually broad and the nose flat. Feet and hands puffy with hands spade-shaped. The child is dull, apathetic, has low body temperature and suffers from constipation and other gastrointestinal complaints. It may be large at birth but as age progresses they have defective development and often stay as dwarfs when they develop into adults. Mentally they range from mildly backward to severely retarded. If diagnosed early enough, iodine or thyroid hormone treatment reverses the condition and in most communities the condition is soon recognized. Only in the more remote areas is it prevalent.

As well as lack of iodine in prenatal or early life, other causes of cretinism are iodide transport defect; failure to convert iodides to the hormones; defective synthesis of thyroglobulin; absent or undeveloped thyroid; failure to respond to thyroid hormones at the cellular level; failure of the gland to respond to thyroid-stimulating hormone (TSH). In all causes, the only treatment is to give oral thyroid hormone, usually thyroxine.

---

cucumber,   a low sodium food that is a good source of potassium and useful amounts of the trace minerals. It contains the following minerals (in mg per 100g): sodium 13; potassium 140; calcium 23; magnesium 9; phosphorus 24; iron 0.3; copper 0.09; zinc 0.1; sulphur 11; chloride 25.

D

---

damsons,   supplies very good intakes of potassium with only small amounts of other minerals. Contents for raw, stewed without and stewed with sugar respectively (in mg per 100g) are: sodium 2, 2, 2; potassium 290, 240, 220; calcium 24, 20, 27; magnesium 11, 10, 9; phosphorus 16, 14, 13; iron 0.4, 0.3, 0.3; copper 0.08, 0.07, 0.05; zinc 0.1, 0.1, 0.1; sulphur 6, 5, 5; chloride trace found in all states.

---

dates,   excellent source of potassium and iron with useful quantities of calcium, magnesium and copper. When dried, edible part supplies the following minerals (in mg per 100g): sodium 5; potassium 750; calcium 68; magnesium 59; phosphorus 64; iron 1.6; copper 0.21; zinc 0.3; sulphur 51; chloride 290.

---

dental caries, a gradual disintegration and dissolution of tooth enamel and dentin that eventually affects the pulp. Results from interaction of three factors: a susceptible tooth surface; acid-forming bacteria; high sugar concentration. Increased intakes of selenium, usually in areas where soil selenium is high, can also induce dental caries in children.

Signs and symptoms include sensitivity to heat and cold; discomfort after eating sugar-based foods; a darkened area between teeth; softened enamel or dentin which becomes obvious on dental examination.

Prevention is a combination of good dental hygiene with adequate intakes of fluoride and calcium. Supplementary fluoride level depends upon concentration of the mineral in the drinking water but a daily total intake up to 1.0mg should be aimed for. Dietary calcium intakes of between 500 and 700mg per day are necessary in children; in adults 800-1000mg calcium may help prevent caries. Children who live in areas of high soil content of molybdenum have low incidence of dental caries so this trace mineral too may prevent the condition developing.

---

dextriferron, iron dextrin injection, provides 100mg iron in 5ml dextriferron solution. May be injected directly into bloodstream. Toxic effects include flushing, nausea, unpleasant taste, headache, abdominal pain and transient diarrhoea. Allergic reactions have been reported. Normally used when oral treatment is ineffective. Total dose of iron in this form over whole treatment should not exceed 2g.

---

diabetes, usually refers to diabetes mellitus, a disorder of carbohydrate metabolism in which sugars in the body are not oxidized to produce energy because of lack of the hormone insulin. Long-term effects include disease changes in both the large and the small blood vessels increasing the chances of atherosclerosis, heart attack, leg ulcers, stroke, kidney failure and blindness (due to diabetic retinopathy). Diabetics tend to lose more zinc in their urine than non-diabetics, suggesting that simple replacement of this by diet or by supplementation can be beneficial. Chromium also tends to be low in the blood of diabetics. This trace mineral is an essential component of glucose tolerance factor which controls blood sugar. Supplementation with this mineral, preferably in the organic form (i.e. in yeast or amino-acid chelated) can also be beneficial. Studies in people suffering from diabetic neuropathy have indicated that their blood magnesium levels are significantly lower than those of people who are not diabetics. Those with the most advanced and severe retinopathy had the lowest blood magnesium levels of all. The significance of these observations is not known but every diabetic should ensure adequate intakes of all three minerals. *See also* glucose tolerance factor.

diabetes insipidus, a disorder induced by lack of production of vasopressin, causing excessive thirst and the production of large volumes of very dilute urine (up to 30 litres per day).

dioctyl sodium sulphosuccinate, a food additive used as an emulsifier and stabilizer; as a wetting agent. Provides 5.2mg sodium per 100mg.

dipotassium hydrogen orthophosphate, also known as dibasic potassium phosphate. E340, used as a food additive as an emulsifying salt; as a buffer. Acceptable daily intake is up to 300mg per kg body weight at normal calcium intakes. Provides 44.8mg potassium and 17.8mg phosphorus per 100mg. Permitted in sterilized and UHT cream; in some cheeses; in condensed milk and dried-milk products; as a permitted miscellaneous additive.

dipotassium tartrate, provides 33.2mg potassium in 100mg tartrate. Used as a saline purgative but must be administered in dilute solution. Acceptable daily intake is up to 105mg potassium tartrate per kg body weight. Usual dose is 2-16g as required. Also allowed as a food additive.

disodium citrate, a food additive used as a buffer; as an emulsifying salt; E331. Acceptable daily intake not limited. Provides 19.5mg sodium per 100mg. Permitted in certain cheeses; in jam and similar products (only for normalizing acidity); as a miscellaneous additive.

disodium dihydrogen diphosphate, also called disodium dihydrogen pyrophosphate; acid sodium pyrophosphate. A food additive, E450a, that functions as a buffer; as a sequestrant; as an emulsifier; as a raising agent for flour; as a colour improver; as a chelating agent. Acceptable daily intake up to 350mg per kg body weight at normal calcium intakes. Provides 13.9mg sodium and 18.8mg phosphorus per 100mg. Permitted in bread; in whipping cream; in some cheeses; in condensed milk and dried-milk products; as a miscellaneous additive.

disodium edetate, also known as EDTA; disodium dihydrogen ethylenediamine-tetra-acetate. A food additive that functions as a sequestrant. Acceptable daily intake up to 2.5mg per kg body weight. Provides 12.4mg sodium per 100mg. Permitted miscellaneous additive; restricted to brandy at 25mg per litre.

disodium tartrate, a food additive, E335, used as a buffer; as an emulsifying salt, as a sequestrant. Acceptable daily intake up to 30mg per kg body weight. Provides 20mg sodium per 100mg. Permitted in some cheeses; as miscellaneous additive; in jam and similar products for controlling acidity.

diuretic drugs, substances that promote the excretion of water and electrolytes by the kidneys. They are used in the treatment of congestive heart failure; liver, kidney or lung diseases that give rise to salt and water retention leading to oedema. The disease process in these conditions is not usually affected by the removal of excess water but the oedema is relieved. Diuretics are used to counter salt and water retention induced by other drug treatments; to enhance the effects of drugs given to reduce high blood pressure; to treat drug overdosage or poisoning to enhance excretion of the toxic materials. The groups of diuretics are:
1. thiazides which inhibit sodium and chloride reabsorption in the kidney and hence promote excretion of these minerals. As a side-effect they also cause excretion of potassium to such an extent that supplementation with the mineral becomes essential; lowered excretion of uric acid which builds up in the joints to cause gout.
2. frusemide type, which act by inhibiting excretion of sodium, potassium and chloride by the kidney, thus increasing water loss. Side-effects as for thiazides.
3. mercurial drugs, which act by inhibiting sodium reabsorption but at different sites in the kidney to other diuretics. Also promote potassium excretion necessitating supplementation with the mineral.

4. aldosterone inhibitors, which function by preventing the action of natural aldosterone. These are potassium-sparing diuretics, decreasing its excretion but promoting that of sodium and chloride. Normally used in conjunction with (1), (2) and (3) above, where they counteract the potassium-losing effects of these diuretics.

5. carbonic anhydrase inhibitors, which act by decreasing the rate of carbonic acid formation and hence acid production. Kidney secretion of acids and reabsorption of bicarbonate and sodium are thereby inhibited. Normally used in conjunction with other diuretics to compensate for increased potassium loss.

6. some diuretics that diminish the excretion of potassium and hence are used with other diuretics to counter their potassium-depleting effects.

7. caffeine, which is a weak diuretic and is found in coffee, tea and other beverages.

8. herbal diuretics which are milder than synthetic drug varieties and are less likely to cause potassium loss.

In addition to potassium loss induced by some of the above diuretics, calcium, magnesium and zinc excretion may also increase under their influence.

---

dolomite,   mixed calcium and magnesium carbonates. Provides 21.7mg calcium and 13.0mg magnesium in 100mg. Usual supplementary dose is 3-6 tablets daily, providing 295 or 591mg calcium and 177 or 354mg magnesium. Taken in the evening, four tablets have been claimed to help induce sleep. Also available as amino-acid chelated dolomite tablets which are claimed to be better absorbed.

---

dried currants,   low sodium food that is rich in potassium and supplying good amounts of calcium, magnesium, iron and copper. Mineral content (in mg per 100g): sodium 20; potassium 710; calcium 95; magnesium 36; phosphorus 40; iron 1.8; copper 0.48; zinc 0.1; sulphur 31; chloride 16.

---

drinking chocolate,   high sodium, potassium, magnesium, phosphorus and iron levels. Good source of copper and zinc. Figures are for the dried form (in mg per 100g): sodium 250; potassium 410; calcium 33; magnesium 150; phosphorus 190; iron 2.4; copper 1.1; zinc 1.9; chloride 130.

---

drinking water, can vary from soft through various grades of hardness. Extent of hardness usually reflects the amount of calcium carbonate in the water but some authorities express water in terms of total dissolved mineral content. Technically a water is regarded as hard if it contains more than 75mg of dissolved solids per litre.

Adults drink on average about 2 litres of water daily and more than half this can be tap water. This quantity in a hard-water area can therefore supply a significant proportion of the daily requirements of minerals — more than 10 per cent of calcium, magnesium, copper, iron and zinc, but all in the ionized inorganic form. A typical daily intake from hard tap water would be (in mg per day): calcium 250; magnesium 50; iron 3; silicon 20; zinc 2; copper 1; fluorine 1 or more; sulphur 0.05; iodine 0.04; chromium 0.01; lithium 0.01; arsenic, lead and mercury — all traces. The benefits of hard water over soft water are from epidemiological studies: lowered mortality rates from cardiovascular disease; a protective effect of calcium in preventing absorption of toxic trace minerals; lower rates of sudden heart failure because of the protective action of the magnesium content; a possible connection between low magnesium rates in tap water and sudden unexpected infant-death syndrome; lower death rates from coronary heart disease related to high silicon content of hard water.

Waters containing significant amounts of fluoride appear also to protect against calcification of the aorta as well as dental caries; iodine from water may contribute up to 20 per cent of daily requirements of the mineral; areas where tap water contains 2.6mg chromium per litre had higher incidence of coronary heart disease than those where the chromium content was 8.6mg per litre; areas where lithium content of tap water is high (8mg per litre) have been reported to have a less aggressive and less competitive population than those where lithium level is low. Other epidemiological studies indicate that in hard water areas there are lower cardiovascular mortality rates, decreased incidence of gastric and duodenal ulcers. Smaller number of admissions for mental diseases and a lower rate of violent behaviour are reported in areas where the drinking water contains 100mg per litre lithium. So many minerals are present in hard water that it is likely that its protective action against heart disease is a result of all being presented together in meaningful amounts. No one has determined with certainty that any one is more significant than another.

Soft water can contain more toxic trace minerals than hard water because it tends to dissolve them from pumping machinery and pipes. All water can be contaminated by industrial effluents like cadmium and mercury or with nitrates from heavily fertilized agricultural land. Water containing high levels of nitrates or nitrites should not be used to make up bottle feeds for babies, since these minerals increase the risk of methaemoglobinaemia, a disease where the blood has a decreased capacity to transport oxygen.

Some waters are so hard that they are partially softened at source before being fed into domestic and industrial water supplies. Domestic softening of water has many advantages for household functions, but the water should be kept separate from that used for drinking. The reasons are twofold:

1. hard water is more conducive to health;
2. the act of softening water with ion exchange resins exchanges the desirable calcium ions for the less desirable sodium ions. Softened water will therefore have an increased sodium content.

---

dripping,   supplies traces only of all the minerals. Beef fat contains the following (in mg per 100g): sodium 5; potassium 4; calcium 1; magnesium trace; phosphorus 13; iron 0.2; sulphur 9; chloride 2.

E

---

eczema,   acute or chronic non-contagious itching, inflammatory disease of the skin.

Some cases respond to oral zinc therapy. Usual dose is 50mg elemental zinc three times daily that can be reduced to 25mg of the mineral three times daily as condition responds. More effective if taken in conjunction with daily vitamin C (1000mg) and essential fatty acids in the form of safflower or oil of evening primrose capsules (three 500mg strength daily). Response can be slow, perhaps needing several months for complete remission.

---

effervescent sodium phosphate,   uses anhydrous sodium phosphate (20 per cent) with sodium bicarbonate, citric acid and tartaric acid. Provides 12.8mg sodium and 21.8mg phosphorus in 100mg mixture. Usual dose is from 4-16g in UK; 10-20g in USA. For uses *see* sodium phosphate, monobasic.

---

eggs, good source of potassium and sodium which is enhanced by salt addition. Calcium content is a useful amount. High in phosphorus and sulphur with significant quantities of iron and zinc.

Quantities for *whole, raw and boiled* (in mg per 100g) are: sodium 140; potassium 140; calcium 52; magnesium 12; phosphorus 220; iron 2.0; copper 0.10; zinc 1.5; sulphur 180; chloride 160.

Fried (in mg per 100g): sodium 220; potassium 180; calcium 64; magnesium 14; phosphorus 260; iron 2.5; copper 0.12; zinc 1.8; sulphur 210; chloride 200.

Poached (in mg per 100g): sodium 110; potassium 120; calcium 52; magnesium 11; phosphorus 240; iron 2.3; copper 0.10; zinc 1.5; sulphur 180; chloride 160.

Omelette (in mg per 100g): sodium 1030; potassium 120; calcium 47; magnesium 18; phosphorus 190; iron 1.7; copper 0.09; zinc 1.3; sulphur 160; chloride 1540.

Scrambled (in mg per 100g): sodium 1050; potassium 130; calcium 60; magnesium 17; phosphorus 190; iron 1.7; copper 0.09; zinc 1.3; sulphur 150; chloride 1580.

---

electrolytes, electrically charged atoms or groups of atoms that exist in aqueous solution. They are known as ions and are divided into anions and cations. *Anions* are negatively charged (so-called because under the influence of an electric current they migrate towards the anode or positive end). Examples are Chloride (Cl^-); phosphate ($PO4^=$); bicarbonate (HCO_3^-) sulphate ($SO_4^=$). *Cations* are positively charged (because under the influence of an electric current they migrate towards the cathode or negative end). Examples are sodium (Na^+); potassium (K^+); calcium (Ca^{++}); magnesium (Mg^{++}). All metals may be regarded as cations when they are present as salts in solution within the body. Hydrogen when positively charged (H^+) confers acidity in solution.

The principle cation inside body cells is potassium (K^+) but magnesium (Mg^{++}) is also present. In fluids that bathe the cells (extracellular fluids) the principle cation is sodium (Na^+), but a small amount of calcium

(Ca^{++}) is also present. Because ions can move freely across cell membranes, the maintenance of potassium inside and sodium outside cells is an energy-requiring process. (*See* sodium pump.) Maintaining this balance is very important to ensure the correct volume of water inside and outside body cells. Imbalance can lead to dehydration or conversely oedema (water retention). All positively charged cations are neutralized by an equal number of negatively charged anions so that the acidity of the fluid of body cells is maintained near neutral.

The transmission of nerve impulses and the contraction of muscles depend upon the correct electrolyte equilibrium at the cell membrane. Whenever a nerve or muscle is active there is a charge of impulse which allows sodium and calcium to enter the appropriate cell; at the same time potassium and magnesium move out of the cell. Once the impulse has passed the ionic pump comes into play to restore the original equilibrium.

The nerves (called motor nerves) that actually stimulate muscle contraction are dependent on the correct calcium-magnesium ionic ratio in the blood. When calcium is lacking these nerves become over-susceptible to stimuli. The result is a condition called tetany, characterized by spasm and twitching of the muscles, particularly those of the face, hands and feet.

Functions of electrolytes are: maintenance of water balance in the body (*see* sodium *and* potassium); maintenance of nerve-impulse transmission; maintenance of smooth muscle contraction; maintenance of acid-alkali (or base) balance of the body (*see* acid-base balance); participation in some enzymatic and hormonal reactions.

The presence of an electrical charge (either positive or negative) on a mineral changes its fundamental properties. *Sodium (Na)* as a pure metal is highly reactive being violently decomposed by water, producing caustic soda and hydrogen which can ignite spontaneously. As the cation sodium (Na^+) it is perfectly stable in water and exists as such in salt solutions and within the body.

Potassium (K) also reacts violently with water, producing caustic potash and hydrogen. As the cation potassion (K^+) it is perfectly stable and exists as such in the body.

Calcium (Ca) reacts with water but less violently than sodium and potassium do. As the cation calcium (Ca^{++}) with two positive charges it is present to a small extent in body fluids as a stable substance necessary for nerve-impulse transmission, muscle contraction and clotting of the blood.

Magnesium (Mg) as the pure metal reacts only very slowly with water and is far more stable than sodium, potassium and magnesium. Heat causes spontaneous ignition with a blinding light which is why it was once used in flash photography. As the cation (Mg^{++}) it carries two positive charges which stabilize the mineral for its functions within the body.

Phosphorus (P) is a very reactive substance that ignites spontaneously at temperatures above 30°C. As the free metal it is highly toxic, causing gastrointestinal irritation, liver damage, skin eruptions, circulatory collapse, coma, convulsions and death with as little as 50mg. On the skin it causes severe burns. When combined with oxygen to form phosphate (PO4) and in its anionic form phosphate ($PO4^{=}$) it is innocuous and performs its functions within the body, as insoluble calcium phosphate in the bones and teeth and as ionic phosphate in body fluids.

Chlorine (Cl) is a highly dangerous, yellow gas with a suffocating odour. As a charged atom chloride (Cl^-) it comprises half of common salt and acts within the body as an important anion that neutralizes the cations sodium and potassium.

---

endive,   a kind of chicory. Main attributes are as a good supplier of potassium and iron. It supplies the following minerals (in mg per 100g): sodium 10; potassium 380; calcium 44; magnesium 10; phosphorus 67; iron 2.8; copper 0.09; sulphur 26; chloride 71.

---

exophthalmia,   abnormal extrusion of the eyeball; pop-eyes. Symptom of Grave's disease due to excessive production of thyroid hormones.

F

---

fatigue,   mental or physical tiredness that may follow prolonged or intense activity; tiredness that cannot be associated with any measurable medical cause. Can produce tearfulness, depression and irritability — the 'housewife syndrome'. Studies indicate that in the absence of any other cause fatigue may be associated with mild deficiency of magnesium and potassium. Supplementation with these minerals is more likely to help in cases of tiredness due to muscle fatigue. Studies indicate that taking extra quantities of magnesium (500mg daily) and potassium (1500mg) daily overcame waking tiredness in a high proportion of individuals suffering from chronic fatigue. Potassium was found to be best taken as increased intakes of fresh fruit and vegetables along with dried fruit and vegetable and fruit juices as part of the diet rather than as tablets. Fatigue caused by lack of iron is associated usually with anaemia. *See* anaemia.

---

fats and oils, usually supply traces only of the minerals, but addition of salt enhances sodium and chloride levels.

Lard contains (in mg per 100g): sodium 2; potassium 1; calcium 1; magnesium 1; phosphorus 3; iron 0.1; copper 0.02; sulphur 25; chloride 4.

Low-fat spread contains (in mg per 100g): traces only of potassium, calcium, magnesium, phosphorus, iron, copper, zinc and sulphur; sodium 690; chloride 1035.

Margarine — all kinds (in mg per 100g): sodium 800; potassium 5; calcium 4; magnesium 1; phosphorus 12; iron 0.3; copper 0.04; sulphur 12; chloride 1200.

Suet in block form contains (in mg per 100g): sodium 21; potassium 13; calcium 6; magnesium 1; phosphorus 7; iron 0.4; copper 0.04; sulphur 20; chloride 18.

Suet as shredded contains traces only of the following minerals: sodium; potassium; calcium; magnesium; phosphorus; iron; copper; zinc; sulphur; chloride.

Vegetable oils also contain traces only of: sodium; potassium; calcium; magnesium; phosphorus; iron; copper; zinc; sulphur; chloride.

---

ferric ammonium citrate, provides 21.5mg iron in 100mg. Daily dose is up to 6.0g total of citrate. It is free of astringent properties and local irritant effect. Usually well tolerated although large doses may cause diarrhoea. Used as a food additive to supply supplementary iron in breadmaking. Permitted miscellaneous additive.

---

ferrocholinate, a chelate prepared from ferric hydroxide and choline dihydrogen citrate. Provides 12.5mg in 100mg. Daily dose for adults is 330-660mg (40-80mg iron) three times daily.

---

ferrous aspartate, provides 14.2mg iron in 100mg. Daily dose of aspartate is 1.0-1.5g with food.

---

ferrous carbonate saccharated, provides 24mg iron in 100mg. Daily dose of carbonate saccharated is 0.6-2.0g with food.

---

ferrous citrate, provides 23.8mg iron in 100mg. Daily dose of citrate is 0.6-2.0g.

---

ferrous fumarate, provides 31.3mg iron in 100mg. Daily dose of fumarate is 200mg (supplementary); 400-600mg (therapeutic). For children up to 1 year, dose is 35mg; 1-5 years, 70mg; 6-12 years, 140mg — all three times daily.

---

ferrous gluconate, provides 12.5 mg iron in 100mg. Daily dose of 600mg (supplementary); 1.2-1.8g (therapeutic). For children aged 6-12 years, dose is 300mg three times daily.

---

ferrous glycine sulphate, also known as ferrous amino-acetosulphate, is a chelate of ferrous sulphate and the amino acid glycine. Provides 17.8mg iron in 100mg. The daily dose is 500-1000mg of ferrous glycine sulphate daily.

---

ferrous lactate, provides 19.4mg iron in 100mg. It is one of the least astringent forms of supplementary iron. Daily dose is 120-600mg of the lactate.

---

ferrous orotate, provides 15.2mg iron in 100mg. Also known as B_{13}-

iron and erroneously as vitamin B_{13}-iron. Has been claimed to be better absorbed than iron salts.

---

ferrous oxalate, provides 31.1mg iron in 100mg. Daily dose is 100-200mg of the oxalate.

---

ferrous succinate, provides 32.6mg iron in 100mg. Daily dose of 200mg succinate (supplementary); 400-600mg (therapeutic). Ferrous succinate is claimed to cause fewer gastrointestinal side-effects than ferrous sulphate.

---

ferrous sulphate, in the crude form is known as green vitriol or green copperas. Provides 20.1mg iron in 100mg. Daily dose 300mg of sulphate (supplementary); 600-900mg (therapeutic). Child's dose is 60mg (1 year), 120mg (1-5 yrs), both three times daily; 300mg (6-12 yrs), twice daily. Therapeutic doses may cause gastrointestinal discomfort, diarrhoea and vomiting. Side-effects occur in 15 per cent of people treated and are related to iron rather than type of preparation. Side-effects are reduced by taking the supplement with or immediately after meals. Continual administration may cause constipation.

Large doses of ferrous sulphate may have irritant and corrosive effects on the lining of the stomach and small intestine and perforation may occur; narrowing of the area may appear later. Symptoms, which may not appear for several hours, include gastric pain, diarrhoea, vomiting and bleeding. Eventually convulsions and coma can occur, leading to liver damage and subsequently death. Treatment must be rapid and includes emetics like 5 per cent sodium bicarbonate as first-line therapy followed by detoxifying drugs under medical supervision. Also used to fortify white flour with iron.

---

ferrous tartrate, provides 22.5mg iron in 100mg. Daily dose is 200-500mg tartrate. Often used when standard iron therapy fails.

---

figs, a low sodium food that is rich in potassium. When dried and cooked supplies enhanced quantities of all minerals. In the raw, green state (in mg per 100g) it supplies: sodium 2; potassium 270; calcium 34; magnesium 20; phosphorus 32; iron 0.4; copper 0.06; zinc 0.3; sulphur 13; chloride 18.

Mineral levels for raw figs, stewed without sugar and stewed with sugar respectively (in mg per 100g) are: sodium 87, 48, 46; potassium 1010, 560, 530; calcium 280, 160, 140; magnesium 92, 51, 48; phosphorus 92, 51, 48; iron 4.2; 2.3, 2.2; copper 0.24, 0.13, 0.13; zinc 0.9, 0.5, 0.5; sulphur 81, 45, 42; chloride 170, 94, 89.

---

fish, should be regarded as a good supplier of sodium, potassium, calcium and phosphorus with significant amounts of iron, copper, zinc and sulphur present. Wide variations depending upon type and cooking additives. Haddock, cod and shrimp supply 100-400µg iodine per 100g; other fish supply from 35-74µg.

White variety includes cod, haddock, halibut, lemon sole, plaice, saithe and whiting. Contents (in mg per 100g) range from: sodium 65-1220; potassium 31-390; calcium 10-110; magnesium 13-35; phosphorus 130-260; iron 0.3-1.8; copper 0.05-0.23; zinc 0.3-1.0; sulphur 130-370; chloride 60-1900.

Fatty fish includes eel, herring, bloater, kipper, mackerel, pilchards, salmon, sardines, sprats, trout, tuna and whitebait. Smoked salmon is the richest source of sodium at 1880mg per 100g. Eel, herring, bloater, kipper, mackerel, pilchards, sardines, sprats, trout, tuna and whitebait supply less (58-990mg per 100g). Whitebait contains the least amount of potassium (110mg per 100g), while the richest source is baked kipper at 520mg per 100g; the other varieties are good sources of potassium ranging from 250-450mg per 100g. Whitebait is richest source of calcium at 860mg per 100g, others supply between 7 and 710mg per 100g. Magnesium content for all fatty fish ranges from 19-52mg per 100g. Richest source of phosphorus is whitebait at 860mg per 100g, others supply 150-640mg per 100g. Low levels of iron in all varieties, ranging from 0.6-5.1mg per 100g. Copper not present in fried herring, bloater, kipper, steamed salmon, sprats, trout and whitebait; others supply low amounts only, from 0.05-0.23. Fried herring, bloater, kipper, steamed salmon, sprats, trout and whitebait do not supply zinc; others have only low quantities, ranging from 0.4-3.0mg per 100g. Sulphur content ranges from 140-310mg per 100g. Richest source of chloride is smoked salmon at 2850mg per 100g; contents for other fatty fish range from 46-1520mg per 100g.

Fish fingers, fried, contain the following (in mg per 100g): sodium 350; potassium 260; calcium 45; magnesium 19; phosphorus 220; iron 0.7; copper 0.08; zinc 0.4; chloride 400.

fluoridation, is the addition of fluoride to a waste water supply that lacks the trace element in order to raise its concentration to a level that will reduce the incidence of dental caries.

It has been known since 1916 that fluoride in drinking water can help prevent dental caries in the teeth of growing children. Since then many epidemiological studies have indicated that where the drinking water contains at least 1mg fluoride per litre water (1 ppm) the incidence of childhood dental caries is lower than in comparable areas where only traces of fluoride are present in the water. The fluorides are believed to be deposited on the enamel surface of developing teeth and this appears to be where they exert their anti-cariogenic action. These observations led to a campaign by various local authorities in the UK to add fluoride to their water supply if this was deficient in fluoride. Western European countries have not accepted fluoridation with the same enthusiasm as Great Britain and many states of the USA, mainly on the grounds that the process is neither safe nor essential.

There seems little doubt from various studies that there is a decline in the incidence of children's dental caries where water previously low in fluorine has had fluoride added to it. What is in doubt is how much this action has contributed to dental health in view of: improvement in dental-health awareness amongst the population as a whole; the knowledge that prevention is possible; better health education; application of fluoridated gel to the teeth of children; mouth rinses containing fluoride; better dental care by the dentist; widespread use of fluoridated toothpaste. Fluoride is now generally accepted as an anti-cariogenic agent — controversy rages over the best way to ensure an adequate intake.

One objection to fluoridation is the possibility of supplying too much fluoride to children and some cases of fluorosis have been noted in those drinking treated water. A more serious objection was raised in the USA where a 5 per cent increase in cancer death-rate in some 20 cities with fluoridated water has not been seriously challenged by fluoridation supporters. The only hard fact to arise from fluoridation of water is that if there are any benefits to be gained, these are confined to a lower incidence of dental caries in children.

Fluorides used to fluoridate drinking water include: hydrofluorosilicic acid; sodium fluoride; sodium silicofluoride.

---

fluorine, chemical symbol F. Atomic weight 19.0. It is a halogen that occurs as fluoride in the earth's crust at an abundance of 65mg per 100g.

Most important natural sources are fluorite, cryolite and florapatite. It is an essential trace element for animals and man.

It was first detected in the animal body by Gay-Lussac in 1805. As fluoride, fluorine is now known to be present in trace amounts in the bones, teeth, thyroid gland and skin of animal and human tissues. When eaten in the food or obtained by drinking water, ingested fluorides are all present as negatively charged atoms (anions) so there is no barrier to absorption. They are rapidly absorbed and distributed in a manner similar to that of chlorides and like these, fluorides tend to stay in the extra-cellular fluid. Much of the fluorides find their way to the skeleton (e.g. in animal studies 60 per cent ended up in the bone after 2 hours), and any excess is efficiently excreted via the urine. Some is also deposited in the teeth but whereas sufficient is protective to the teeth, excess can be harmful. Blood levels of fluoride are between 14 and 19μg per 100ml, of which 15-20 per cent is ionic. The mineral does not appear to cross the barrier from blood plasma to breast milk, so increasing maternal intakes during lactation is unlikely to provide more for the baby. More fluoride is retained by the body during childhood than in the adult state.

Food sources of fluoride are widespread and drinking water supplies appreciable amounts. Few quantitative analyses of individual foods for the mineral are available, but the UK Ministry of Agriculture, Food and Fisheries has published the following average intakes (in mg per day): cereals 0.15; meat 0.05; fish 0.08; fats 0.03; fruits and sugars 0.04; root vegetables 0.04; other vegetables 0.02; milk 0.09, and beverages (not including fluoride from the water source) 1.33.

Total dietary intake is thus estimated at 1.82mg fluoride per day. To this must be added the amount contained in the water supply. Assuming an intake of 1.1 litres daily, unfluoridated water will supply an extra 0.11-0.21mg; fluoridated water will supply 1.1mg extra fluoride. The richest source of dietary fluoride is tea, particularly the China variety which contains up to 10mg fluoride in 100g dried leaves. Six cups of this daily will provide about 3mg fluoride from the infused dried leaves alone. Indian tea will provide about half this quantity.

Functions of fluoride are not known with certainty, but it appears to confer strength and stability to bones and teeth, probably by forming insoluble fluoro-phosphates; it acts as an anti-cariogenic agent in the developing teeth of children, probably by reducing the solubility of tooth minerals or by discouraging the growth of acid-producing bacteria in the mouth; it may play a part in preventing osteoporosis in the elderly.

Deficiency in animals causes anaemia in mice; infertility in mice; stunted growth in rats and chicks; lack of skeletal development in rats and chicks. In human beings, deficiency gives rise to dental caries in children; osteoporosis in elderly adults (possibly) where it may be associated with low calcium intakes.

Signs of deficiency are probably confined to the appearance of caries in the teeth of children. *See* dental caries.

Therapy of deficiency can be: fluoridation of drinking water supplies, *see* fluoridation; use of fluoride toothpaste; oral fluoride tablets; direct application to teeth of fluoride gel; mouth rinses with fluoride solutions. All have been claimed to be effective in reducing the incidence of dental caries in children.

Therapy: sodium fluoride has been used to treat osteoporosis; Paget's disease; bone pain; otosclerosis. (See entries under specific complaint.)

Excessive intakes of fluoride causes fluorosis.

In cattle and sheep excessive intakes may be taken when they graze on land contaminated with fluoride-containing dust. Both teeth and skeleton are affected. Signs are first seen in the teeth of young, growing animals as white mottled patches and a rough enamel surface. In adult animals the surfaces of the large bones and lower jaw become thickened and the bone density thickens with extra calcification. Sometimes bony outgrowths appear. Weakness and reduced milk yield are also signs of excessive fluoride intake in dairy animals.

In man, the first and most obvious sign is mottling of the teeth caused when the chalky-white irregular patches on the surface of the enamel become infiltrated by yellow or brown staining. Severe fluorosis weakens the enamel, resulting in surface pitting. All teeth may be affected but fluorosis is seen on the incisors of the upper jaw. Dental fluorosis does not mean that skeletal fluorosis is present, but the latter can occur with extremely high intakes of fluoride taken over long periods.

When the water supply contains more than 10mg fluoride per litre of water (10 ppm) or when excessive amounts of fluoride are inhaled as in smelting aluminium, fluorosis affects more than the teeth. Appetite is depressed; there is increased density (sclerosis) of the bones of the spine, pelvis and limbs; the supple ligaments of the spine become calcified; resulting in the so-called 'poker back'; calcium is deposited in muscles and tendons; nerve disturbances following the changes in the spinal column can appear. All of these changes are classed as osteosclerosis.

Treatment of fluorosis is to reduce the intake of dietary fluoride.

Recommended dietary intake of fluoride is suggested as 1mg per day in adults by the West German authorities. The Dental Health Committee of the British Dental Association has recommended intakes of fluoride (in mg per day) as: 2 weeks to 2 yrs 0.25; 2-4 yrs 0.5; 4-16 yrs 1.0. This advice applies where water fluoride levels are below 0.3mg per litre. When the water fluoride level is between 0.3 and 0.7mg per litre, no supplements should be given until age 2 years, after which doses are halved.

The ideal drinking water supply is regarded as 1mg per litre, which would supply between 1 and 2mg fluoride daily. Whilst this may be suitable for growing children who drink milk, which has very little fluoride content, it is additive for those who drink tea which is rich in the mineral.

---

fluorosis,   excessive deposition of fluoride in the teeth causing mottling. Can also apply to large amounts of fluoride deposited in bone. *See* fluorine.

---

food sources,   a balanced diet will provide trace minerals from all food items and a major study has indicated the contributions made by such ingredients to the daily requirements. These average intakes of trace minerals were obtained from the 'total diet study' by chemical analysis of food. Representative amounts of 68 foods (based on National Food Survey information to include sweets, water and soft drinks) were obtained, prepared, cooked then analysed. The results are as shown in Table 3.

Table 3: Trace minerals obtained from an average balanced diet

Foodstuffs	Zinc (mg)	Copper (mg)	Iodine (µg)	Selenium (mg)	Manganese (mg)	Fluoride (mg)
Cereals	1.8	0.38	31	30	1.42	0.16
Meat and eggs	3.5	0.37	36	12	0.08	0.05
Fish	0.1	0.03	15	10	0.01	0.07
Milk	1.5	0.04	92	4	0.04	0.03
Fats/dairy products	0.9	0.02	17	1	0.16	0.03
Root vegetables	0.6	0.16	15	1	0.22	0.02
Other vegetables	0.3	0.10	8	1	0.17	0.01
Fruit and sugar products	0.4	0.20	25	1	0.20	0.04
Beverages	0.3	0.17	16	0	2.92	1.41
TOTAL	9.4	1.47	255	60	5.08	1.82

The sources of iron in the diet have been calculated by a similar method as well from a national food survey (see Table 4). With this method there is a continuous survey of 7500 randomly elected households throughout Britain each year. The person responsible for food records the type, amount and cost of each item brought into the home. Alcoholic drinks and sweets are left out. Meals and snacks eaten outside the home are also excluded. Take-away meals, picnics and lunches made from the household food supply are included. Calcium and iron are routinely evaluated but zinc, copper and manganese intakes are sometimes assessed.

Table 4: Contributions of major groups of foods to iron intakes

Foodstuff	National Food Survey		Total Diet Study	
	mg per day	per cent	mg per day	per cent
Cereals	4.1	37	5.1	45
Meat and eggs	3.1	29	2.8	25
Fish	0.2	2	0.2	2
Milk	0.2	2	0.4	4
Fats/dairy products	0.2	2	0.1	1
Root vegetables	0.8	7	0.8	7
Other vegetables	1.1	11	0.9	8
Fruit and sugar products	0.6	5	0.7	6
Beverages	0.1	1	0.2	2
Other foods	0.5	4	—	—
TOTAL	10.9	100	11.2	100

The National Food Survey method allows contributions of iron from individual foods as well as from food groups to be estimated. For example, of the 11mg iron in the diet, 1.1mg was derived from food fortification (mainly from white flour); 1.3mg was haem iron; 8.6mg was natural non-haem iron. Other minerals will be evaluated eventually in a similar manner.

French beans, supply significant quantities of potassium, calcium and the trace minerals. When boiled, minerals contained (in mg per 100g): are sodium 3; potassium 100; calcium 39; magnesium 10; phosphorus 15; iron 0.6: copper 0.10; zinc, 0.3; sulphur 8; chloride 11.

fruit pie filling, supplies all the minerals with useful quantities of potassium and iron. Canned, it supplies the following minerals (in mg per 100g): sodium 30; potassium 79; calcium 18; magnesium 4; phosphorus 9; iron 0.5; copper 0.03; zinc 0.1; chloride 45.

---

fruit salad, good source of potassium and iron with only traces of sodium. Canned fruit salad contains (in mg per 100g): sodium 2; potassium 120; calcium 8; magnesium 8; phosphorus 10; iron 1.0; copper 0.03; sulphur 2; chloride 3.

G

---

geophagia, also known as clay eating. The habit of eating clay is common in rural areas of the United States, in the Middle East and in some areas of Africa. The practice is considered normal during pregnancy in many places throughout the world, usually amongst communities in the lower economic strata, and is believed to supply calcium. Clay is eaten for its mineral content; to relieve hunger; to relieve gastrointestinal discomfort; to overcome diarrhoea; to detoxify harmful minerals. Amongst people on poor diets, clay eating can provide substantial quantities of essential minerals. There is no evidence that the practice causes ill-effects, but once diets are improved, the habit usually stops. It has been associated also with an attempt to cure iron deficiency by some researchers; others believe that geophagia causes malabsorption of iron inducing anaemia. Zinc too is supplied in clay, but the chelating effect of clay on zinc may make it unavailable and at the same time immobilize zinc from other dietary sources.

---

glucose tolerance factor, usually abbreviated to GTF, is the only active form of chromium known to function in the body. It is present in foods and can be synthesized in the body from trivalent chromium, nicotinic acid and certain amino acids. It is a complex whose exact structure is not known, so only natural source material is available.

Its history goes back to 1929 when yeast extracts were found to potentiate the action of the hormone insulin. This action was attributed to the vitamins in yeast, and interest waned until 1955 when rats fed on torula yeast were found to develop diabetes and liver degeneration. No known nutrients were able to reverse these conditions so the existence of a new dietary agent, GTF, was postulated. In the early 1960s GTF was identified as a complex of trivalent chromium, nicotinic acid and protein-like material. Animals fed diets deficient in the complex developed a diabetes-like condition.

In the mid-1960s many adults and elderly people with glucose intolerance (a factor in diabetes) were found to improve on a supplement of 150-250µg chromium daily in the form of chromic chloride. Similar benefits were noted in malnourished children in Jordan, Nigeria and Turkey, but not from Egypt. This suggested that children in Egypt, unlike the others, did not lack chromium. Many experiments and observations then led to the conclusions that:

1. simple chromium salts did not meet the criteria of an essential element;
2. chromium salts did not cross the placental barrier;
3. chromium salts supplementation in man always took several days or weeks to be noticeable;
4. chromium salts did not equilibrate with body pool of organic chromium;
5. calculations of chromium balance in man indicated a very wide deficit when the absorption rate for chromic chloride was assumed to be the same as for food chromium. For example, if food chromium were absorbed at the same rate as chromic chloride, its calculated dietary intake of 50-100µg per day would lead to only 0.25-0.5µg in the urine. The usual daily excretion via this route is 7-10µg, suggesting that more food-origin chromium is absorbed and more excreted.

Chromium in the form of brewer's yeast is better absorbed, can be transported across the placenta, is quickly distributed to the tissues and has a faster action in reducing blood sugar than does chromic chloride in rat experiments. Studies in isolating the factor thus yielded GTF, albeit in a crude form.

GTF is far superior to chromium salts as a therapeutic or supplementary form of chromium. Attempts to synthesize it from chromium, nicotinic acid and amino acids have not been successful. Twenty-five per cent of the chromium of GTF in brewer's yeast is absorbed compared with 1 per cent of chromium salts. Yeast can be enriched with chromium by adding the mineral salt to growing yeast, removing the excess chromium salt and drying the yeast. In this way yeast is available containing up to 60µg chromium per g of yeast, all of it presented as GTF. Although precise quantitative assessment of GTF is difficult, the following foods are known to be rich in it (all in descending order of biological activity): dried brewer's yeast; black pepper; calves' liver; cheese; wheatgerm. Moderate sources are: wholemeal bread; cornflakes; white bread; spaghetti; beef; wholewheat grain; butter; rye bread; margarine; oysters; chilli peppers; wheat bran; shrimp. Poorer, but nonetheless useful, sources are: lobster; mushrooms; chicken leg; haddock; beer; egg-white; chicken breast; skimmed milk.

The toxicity of GTF is low. Studies suggest that human beings can tolerate up to 1mg per kg body weight or 60mg in the average adult. The corresponding figure for chromium salts is 18mg.

---

glycerophosphates, introduced into medicine on the grounds that lecithin contains phosphorus in the form of glycerophosphate and therefore these compounds would be more easily assimilated into body tissues and particularly the brain. No evidence to support this but glycerophosphates were widely used in the past and are still used as general tonics rather than as suppliers of phosphorus.

---

goitre, a swelling of the neck due to enlargement of the thyroid gland — the gland enlarges in an attempt to increase the output of hormone.

Endemic is goitre due to lack of iodine in the soil and hence in the diet.

Sporadic is due usually to simple overgrowth of the gland or to a tumour.

Exophthalmic is when the swelling is associated with overactivity of the gland. *See* Grave's disease. The condition may also be due to increased intake of certain foods. *See* goitrogens.

Goitres are particularly apt to occur at puberty and during pregnancy.

Endemic goitre occurs mainly in three types of terrain:

1. mountainous areas of Europe, Asia, North and South America, the Alps, Himalayas, Andes, Rockies, Cameroon mountains, Highlands of New Guinea;

2. on alluvial plains once covered by glaciers, e.g., the area around the Great Lakes of North America, some areas of New Zealand;

3. in isolated localities where the water originates in limestone, e.g., Derbyshire and the Cotswolds of England. Simple goitres in non-endemic areas also occur, e.g., in Glasgow where iodine intake was found to be only 60 per cent of the norm.

Treatment of endemic goitre with iodine has been known since the mid-eighteenth century, but it was not until 1920 that American researchers D. Marine and O. P. Kimball demonstrated unequivocally that sodium iodide reduced the incidence of goitre in children. Confirmation of the presence of thyroxine in the thyroid gland came from E. C. Kendall and A. E. Osterberg of the USA in 1919; that of triiodothyronine came from J. Gross and R. Pitt-Rivers of the UK in 1952.

Endemic goitre responds to iodide therapy. Simple goitre in non-endemic areas rarely requires treatment. Iodides are unlikely to cause it to shrink. Only if the goitre becomes disfiguring is thyroxine used. If this is unsuccessful surgery is usually considered. When the goitre is due to intakes of goitrogenic foods, these should be discontinued.

---

goitrogens, substances found in some foods that inhibit formation of hormones by the thyroid gland. They occur principally in the seeds of cabbage, mustard and rape and also in cabbage leaves, kale and turnips. The active substances are glucosinolates and thiocyanates which prevent the synthesis of thyroxine and reduce the amount of iodine in the thyroid gland respectively. There is no strong evidence that these foods cause goitre in man — probably because not enough is eaten. It is possible in farm animals who have large intakes of these foods and some of the goitrogens may find their way into the milk but not enough to cause goitre in the humans who drink it. Ground-nuts, cassava and soya beans are also goitrogenic but the active principles are not known. Cooking methods tend to destroy goitrogens.

---

gold, chemical symbol Au from the Latin *aurum*. Atomic weight 197. A food additive used in the form of gold leaf as a colour for external decoration. Acceptable daily intake has not been allocated as its use is very limited and not considered a hazard. Permitted colouring matter that is restricted to external application, to dragées and sugar-coated confectionery. For medicinal uses of gold *see* gold salts.

---

gold salts, gold thioglucose; sodium aurothiomalate; sodium aurothiosulphate. All are used in treating rheumatoid arthritis. Ineffective in osteoarthritis. Given by deep intramuscular injection, either in aqueous solution or in oil suspension. Toxic effects include mouth ulceration; itching; urticaria; eczema; seborrheic dermatitis; alopecia; inflamed gums;

gastritis; colitis. Skin reactions are the most common. Blood abnormalities and kidney damage may also occur.

---

golden syrup, good source of iron with high quantities of both sodium and potassium. Supplies minerals (in mg per 100g): in the following levels: sodium 270; potassium 240; calcium 26; magnesium 10; phosphorus 20; iron 1.5; copper 0.09; sulphur 54; chloride 42.

---

gooseberries, almost sodium free, the food contributes good amounts of potassium with small amounts of the trace minerals. Levels of the following minerals (in mg per 100g) are for green raw and ripe raw respectively: sodium 2, 1; potassium 210, 170; calcium 28, 19; magnesium 7, 9; phosphorus 34, 19; iron 0.3, 0.6; copper 0.13, 0.15; zinc 0.1, 0.1; sulphur 16, 14; chloride 7, 11.

Green variety, stewed without sugar and with sugar respectively (in mg per 100g) contains: sodium 2, 2; potassium 180, 160; calcium 24, 22; magnesium, 6, 5; phosphorus 29, 27; iron 0.3, 0.2; copper 0.11, 0.10; zinc 0.1, 0.1; sulphur 14, 13; chloride 6, 5.

---

grapefruit, a low sodium food that is a good provider of potassium, particularly in the raw state. When canned, all levels are reduced because of dilution with syrup. Mineral levels for raw and canned variety respectively (in mg per 100g) are: sodium 1, 10; potassium 230, 79; calcium 17, 17; magnesium 10, 7; phosphorus 16, 13; iron 0.3, 0.7; copper 0.06, 0.03; zinc 0.1, 0.4; sulphur 5, 0; chloride 1, 5.

---

grapefruit juice, an important source of potassium that is virtually sodium free but containing only small amounts of other minerals. As canned for unsweetened and sweetened, mineral levels of the following are identical (in mg per 100g): potassium 110; calcium 9; phosphorus 12; iron 0.3; copper 0.03; chloride 10. Only slight differences occur between unsweetened and sweetened for the following: sodium 3, 2; magnesium 8, 9 and zinc 0.4, 0.3.

---

grapes, virtually sodium free and supplying significant amounts of potassium. Small amounts of all other minerals present. Black raw and white raw respectively (in mg per 100g) contain: sodium 2, 2; potassium 320, 250; calcium 4, 19; magnesium, 4, 7; phosphorus 16, 22; iron 0.3, 0.3; copper 0.08, 0.10; zinc 0.1, 0.1; sulphur 7, 9; chloride traces only present in both varieties.

Grave's disease, *see* hyperthyroidism.

greengages, sodium-free food whose main mineral component is potassium, but small amounts of all other minerals present. Quantities of minerals (in mg per 100g) for raw, stewed without sugar and stewed with sugar respectively, are: sodium, identical in all three states, 1; potassium 310, 260, 240; calcium 17, 15, 13; magnesium 8, 6, 5; phosphorus 23, 20, 18; iron 0.4, 0.3, 0.3; copper 0.08, 0.07, 0.06; zinc, identical level of 0.1; sulphur 3, 3, 2; chloride, identical in all three forms, 1.

guavas, low sodium food providing useful quantity of potassium with small amounts of other minerals. Figures are available only for canned fruit (in mg per 100g): sodium 7; potassium 120; calcium 8; magnesium 6; phosphorus 11; iron 0.5; copper 0.10; zinc 0.4; chloride 10.

gum disease, also known as periodontal disease, characterized by a progressive inflammation and infection of the gum tissue and underlying jaw-bone. Believed to be due to residual food, bacteria and tartar deposits that collect in the tiny crevices between the gums and the necks of the teeth. As the bacterial infection spreads deeper into the tissue surrounding the jaw-tooth connection, the gums recede until teeth loosen and fall out. Resistance to gum disease may be increased with correct diet. Extra calcium has been shown to reduce the onset of the complaint and in some cases reverse it. Typical intakes were 500mg calcium twice daily. Found to be important at the same time to maintain low dietary phosphorus:calcium ratio. Ideal ratio is 1:1 but most popular foods have a high ratio, e.g., meat 20:1; refined cereals 6:1; potatoes 5:1. Soft drinks are high in phosphorus. Bonemeal has 1:2 ratio but since much phosphorus is supplied in other foods, the ideal calcium supplement for periodental disease is that with no phosphorus. Dolomite, amino-acid chelated calcium, calcium gluconate, calcium lactate and calcium orotate are all suitable.

H

hair analysis, assay of a sample of hair for its mineral content. After preparation and dissolution of the hair, the resulting liquid is measured for minerals using atomic absorption spectroscopy; neutron activation analysis or electron microprobe analysis allowing accurate determinations of many trace minerals at concentrations down to $0.1\mu g$ per gram and less in some cases. Hair analysis offers certain advantages over the more usual blood and urine analysis for minerals. These are:

1. hair provides a better assessment of normal trace mineral concentrations because these reflect average levels over the period of growth;

2. hair allows long-term variations in trace mineral concentrations to be assessed. As hair grows, it reflects body status of minerals during the period of growth so if long hair is subdivided into lengths, measurement will show the variation in mineral content over those periods. The technique has been used to determine mineral status during pregnancy.

3. hair is an inert, chemically homogeneous substance that is a permanent record of the minerals in it. Once a mineral has been deposited in hair it stays there.

4. the concentrations of most trace elements are higher in hair than those in blood and most tissues of the body. Chromium levels are 50 times higher in hair than in blood; cobalt levels are 100 times higher.

5. hair provides a record of past as well as recent trace-mineral levels. Body status can therefore be measured in retrospect.

6. collection of hair is painless, is not an invasive technique, can be carried out by unqualified persons and the product can be kept indefinitely without deterioration.

Against the value of hair analysis are the objections that:

1. there is a possibility of variations across the scalp. Any variation can be minimized by taking hair always from the same part of the head, usually the short hair at the back.

2. procedures for washing and preparing the hair sample before analysis can differ amongst those carrying out the assays. The washing stage can be with solvents or with detergents but studies suggest that the two are compatible and the problem is not serious.

3. hair may have been treated with bleach or dye which can leach out

trace elements. Shampooing and conditioning do not have this effect.

4. zinc and selenium are used extensively in hair shampoos, colouring agents and conditioners and these may be absorbed into the hair. There is no clear evidence that this happens.

5. there is no correlation between concentrations of trace elements in hair and in blood. This is not surprising in view of the differing time-scales that each type of assay reflects. Comparative hair analyses carried out by the same procedures by the same analyst on the same individual over a particular time-scale could give useful information about body changes in mineral status.

Interpretation of hair analysis is not straightforward and should be left to an expert. It has been suggested that hair examination in this way is of more use in determining toxic minerals and the significance of levels of essential minerals is debatable. There do appear to be correlations between low levels of hair copper and high levels of hair zinc with higher blood pressure in man. There is strong positive correlation between some toxic elements in hair and the incidence of high blood pressure in children. Low hair-zinc levels are known to be associated with dwarfism. It has also been claimed that certain patterns are emerging, for example that:

1. schizophrenics have high calcium, low iron, high copper and low zinc levels in their hair;

2. arthritics have high lead, low iron and low copper levels in their hair. Sometimes they show low manganese and a high calcium level that may depress magnesium concentration.

3. diabetics often have low chromium, low manganese and low zinc with excessively high calcium levels in their hair. The significance of these findings has not yet been worked out. They cannot be regarded as diagnostic of these conditions without accompanying biochemical analyses and clinical signs.

For most individuals it is safe to treat low levels of essential minerals in hair with a change in diet or supplements to supply those minerals that are low. Essential minerals that are present in high quantity may then be reduced to normal levels. High levels of toxic minerals should be treated by a qualified practitioner who will assess their significance by carrying out other tests. High calcium intakes combined with vitamin C and pectin is one combination that may help remove small amounts of toxic trace minerals.

---

haricot beans, excellent source of iron, zinc and copper trace minerals.

A low sodium food that is an important source of potassium, calcium, magnesium, phosphorus and sulphur. Levels of minerals present for raw and boiled respectively (in mg per 100g) are: sodium 43, 15; potassium 1160, 320; calcium 180, 65; magnesium 180, 45; phosphorus 310, 120; iron 6.7, 2.5; copper 0.61, 0.14; zinc 2.8, 1.0; sulphur 170, 46; chloride 2, 1.

Hashimoto's disease, also known as Hashimoto's thyroiditis; Hashimoto's struma; chronic lymphatic thyroiditis; auto-immune thyroiditis. The most common cause of hypothyroidism. More prevalent in women (8 times as often as in men) and usually between the ages of 30 and 50 years. It is an auto-immune disorder where the body produces disordered immunological response against itself to such an extent as to cause tissue injury.

Symptoms are painless enlargement of the thyroid gland or a feeling of fullness in the throat.

Treatment is that for myxoedema (*see* myxoedema).

---

hazel nuts, sodium-free food supplying important dietary levels of iron, copper and zinc. Useful calcium, magnesium, phosphorus and sulphur levels. Also known as cob nuts, they contain levels of the following minerals (in mg per 100g): sodium 1; potassium 350; calcium 44; magnesium 56; phosphorus 230; iron 1.1; copper 0.21; zinc 2.4; sulphur 75; chloride 6.

---

heart disease, adequate intakes of certain minerals appear from epidemiological and other studies to protect against heart disease and in some cases can benefit the individual with the complaint. The minerals are:
1. calcium and magnesium, where observations suggest that those communities living in hard-water areas have fewer cases of heart disease than those living in soft-water areas. Hard water contains many minerals, but the main ones are calcium and magnesium and these are believed to exert a protective effect.
2. calcium, which in adequate quantities tends to reduce blood-cholesterol levels. Low body-calcium levels result in high blood-cholesterol levels. Calcium may act in the intestine by combining with fatty acids to form insoluble calcium soaps that are excreted. This reduces fat absorption and lowers blood fats. Both fats and cholesterol levels can be reduced with intakes of calcium between 1025 and 1200mg per day. The mineral appears

to function by reducing LDL (low-density lipoprotein) cholesterol levels but allows HDL (high-density lipoprotein) cholesterol levels to be maintained. The end-result is reduction in the severity of atherosclerosis.

3. magnesium, which in adequate quantities appears to prevent cardiac spasms. Post-mortem studies on those who have died from heart disease indicate lower heart-muscle levels of magnesium than in those who have died of other causes. Magnesium is believed to dilate blood vessels in the heart; calcium causes constriction. Correct balance of both minerals ensures the heart beats smoothly. When magnesium is short the imbalance can cause constriction which in turn gives rise to cardiac spasm. Diet and supplementation should ensure adequate intakes of both minerals.

4. potassium, which helps to counteract the negative effects of sodium on the blood pressure. Post-mortem studies indicate that in those dying suddenly from heart attacks, potassium levels in the heart muscle are also low. Low potassium concentration is associated with angina. Low magnesium and potassium levels may be localized because of heart problems (rather than causing them) but sensible insurance against heart attacks is adequate intakes of potassium as well as the other minerals.

5. selenium, which when deficient in animals gives rise to heart problems and high blood pressure. In human studies, those who live in areas where soil selenium and hence selenium intakes are low have the highest rates of coronary disease. Where selenium intakes are highest, rates of coronary disease are lowest. The largest trial was in China, involving more than 45,000 people, in an area where selenium is low. In this area heart disease is rife, affecting many of the population; supplementation with selenium in thousands of children reduced the rate of heart disease from 40 per 1000 to zero. The death-rate in those already afflicted was reduced from 50 per cent to 6 per cent simply by feeding small amounts of selenium (200μg per day). *See* Keshan disease.

6. chromium, which is usually low in the heart tissues of those dying from heart disease. Chromium appears to play a significant role in increasing the highly desirable HDL cholesterol levels at the expense of the less desired LDL cholesterol levels. This alone will help reduce the chances of development of heart failure.

7. manganese, which has been found in low concentration in the heart tissue of those dying from cardiac problems.

---

high blood pressure, may be associated with high sodium, low potassium, high cadmium intakes. *See* heart disease; salt. High cadmium intakes antagonize the uptake and metabolism of selenium in the body so the effect of this toxic mineral may be mediated through these effects or in a direct action of its own.

---

honeycomb, poor source of most minerals apart from potassium and phosphorus. Mineral figures (in mg per 100g) are: sodium 7; potassium 35; calcium 8; magnesium 2; phosphorus 32; iron 0.2; copper 0.04; sulphur 1; chloride 26.

---

hydrochloric acid, a mineral acid, produced by the parietal cells of the stomach, that provides the acidic medium of the gastric juices needed for the early stages of food digestion. Gastric juice contains between 0.2 and 0.5 per cent hydrochloric acid. The acid is a combination of hydrogen ions (which determine acidity) and chloride ions. Hydrogen ions arise by the dissociation of carbonic acid, itself produced from carbon dioxide and water in the blood. Carbonic acid production is under the control of an enzyme carbonic anhydrase which contains zinc. Only the hydrogen ions from the dissociation of carbonic acid pass from the blood to the parietal cells of the stomach (bicarbonate ions are unable to do so), where they combine with the readily available chloride ions to form hydrochloric acid.

Excessive production of hydrochloric acid causes heartburn, gastric and duodenal ulcers.

Deficiency of hydrochloric acid production (known as hypochloryhdria) or complete lack (known as achlorhydria) can lead to malabsorption of some minerals that are usually solubilized by hydrochloric acid; chronic gastritis due to destruction of the parietal cells. The condition is associated with pernicious anaemia; gastric cancer and other cancers of the gastrointestinal tract possibly because in the absence of hydrochloric acid certain cancer-forming substances can be produced from normal food ingredients.

Supplementary forms of hydrochloric acid are:
1. dilute hydrochloric acid. Two to five ml of 10 per cent hydrochloric acid are diluted with 200-250ml of water and sipped through a straw during the course of a meal. No more than 20ml of the 10 per cent hydrochloric acid should be taken over 24 hours.
2. betain hydrochloride, which provides 23.8mg hydrochloric acid in 100mg. Usual dose is 60-500mg dissolved in water which is drunk after meals. Also available in tablet form.

3.   glutamic acid hydrochloride, which provides 19.9mg hydrochloric acid in 100mg. Usual dose is 600-1800mg which is dissolved in water and drunk after meals. Also available in tablet and capsule forms.

---

hydrofluorsilicic acid,   provides 13.2mg fluoride in 100mg acid. Used in controlled amounts for the fluoridation of drinking water.

---

hyperthyroidism,   also known as thyrotoxicosis; Grave's disease; Basedow's disease; Plummer's disease; toxic diffuse goitre; toxic modular goitre. Characterized by an excessive secretion of thyroid gland hormones which increase the metabolic rate.

All forms of hyperthyroidism give rise to the following signs and symptoms: goitre; fast heartbeat; warm, fine, moist skin; tremor; eye signs that include stare, lid lag, lid retraction, eye pain, excessive tears, irritation, sensitivity to light; nervousness; increased activity; increased sweating; heart sensitivity; palpitations; fatigue; increased appetite; weight loss; insomnia; weakness; excessive bowel movements sometimes leading to diarrhoea. In addition symptoms confined to Grave's disease include abnormal extrusion of the eyeball (exophthalmia) and an itchy, red, coarse and thick skin.

Treatment consists of:
1.   iodine in high doses usually in the form of potassium iodide or sodium iodide, orally or by intravenous injection. Lasts only up to a week and functions by inhibiting incorporation of iodine into thyroid hormones.
2.   antithyroid drugs that inhibit the incorporation of iodine into thyroid hormones;
3.   radioactive iodine, used in female patients past their child-bearing years and in males. No evidence of increased incidence of tumours, leukaemia or cancer of the thyroid after this treatment. Therapy of choice in those above 40 years of age with Grave's disease.
4.   surgery, in all age groups, to remove the whole or part of the thyroid. Sometimes hypothyroidism occurs and can be treated with thyroxine. After complete removal of the thyroid, thyroxine therapy is needed for life.

---

hypothyroidism,   *see* cretinism; Hashimoto's disease; myxoedema.

I

impotence, inability of the male to attain or sustain an erection satisfactorily for normal sexual intercourse. Noted in patients undergoing kidney dialysis who were found to have low blood levels of zinc because the dialysing fluids lacked the mineral. Remedying this restored normal sexual function. Earlier studies on zinc deficient populations in the Middle East and elsewhere found that lack of dietary zinc gave rise to retarded sexual development in growing children. Increasing zinc intakes allowed normal development to continue. Zinc has been shown to help in some cases of sexual dysfunction in adult males. Low testosterone (male sex hormone) levels were associated with low blood-zinc concentration resulting in low sperm counts. Increasing dietary zinc from the food and by supplementing with 30mg of the mineral daily restored sexual function to normal.

Indian childhood cirrhosis, a rapidly progressive disorder and an important cause of death in the Asian subcontinent. Characterized by excessive copper deposits in the liver and kidneys of children affected. Earlier onset than Wilson's disease but treatment is similar (*See* Wilson's disease).

intra-uterine devices, known also as the coil or IUD. Copper has been known to be toxic to spermatozoa since the mid-eighteenth century and the metal is incorporated into intra-uterine devices. A typical copper T-shaped IUD has a copper surface of 135 square millimetres and releases about 29µg of copper daily into the uterine fluid. Localized high concentration of the mineral is believed sufficient to cause a contraceptive effect although local irritations by the device may also play a part. The end-result is inhibition of implantation of the fertilized ovum.

iodine, chemical symbol I. Atomic weight 126.9. A halogen that is an essential trace element. Abundance in igneous rocks is 300µg per kg; in sea water 0.5µg per litre.

Distribution of iodine throughout the world is extremely variable. Areas that lack the mineral in the soil are described as the 'goitre belt' since goitre is the most prevalent disease caused by deficiency of iodine. In the United States there is a wide belt across the middle of the country stretching from east to west; in the UK the Midlands and south-west England soils lack iodine and the disease was once common, hence the popular name for goitre was 'Derbyshire neck'. Vast tracts of China and large areas of Africa, continental Europe, Russia and South America are all classed as 'goitre belts'. Fresh water provides only small amounts of iodine (in Britain from $1-50\mu g$ per litre) and this level provides a guide to the soil which the water irrigates. Low levels in the soil are reflected in the fruit and vegetables grown in that soil. Those who live in and eat exclusively the produce from an iodine-deficient area have a greater chance of developing goitre. Now that most diets are composed of food from a variety of areas, such deficiency is more rare. In the soil, in the diet and to a large extent in the body, iodine exists in the form of iodide.

Body content of iodine in adults is between 20 and 50mg. Most of this is concentrated in the thyroid gland situated in the base of the neck. All vertebrate animals need iodine and all possess a thyroid gland or tissue in some part of the body. Any iodine in the diet is quickly absorbed from the intestinal tract, mostly in the form of iodide. It is rapidly transported in the blood to the thyroid gland where it is stored before conversion into the thyroid hormones. These are released as required. The amount of iodide taken into thyroid depends upon the activity of the gland.

In the thyroid, iodide is oxidized to iodine which is combined with the amino acid tyrosine to produce mono- and di-iodotyrosines. Further conversion of these to the hormones triiodothyronine (T3) and thyroxine (T4) takes place in the epithelial cells of the gland. Both hormones are stored as thyroglobulin, a complex with the protein globulin. Once released, the hormones are carried in the blood loosely bound to an alpha-globulin. Normal values of thyroxine and triiodothyronine in blood serum are between 4 and $11\mu g$ and between 70 and $190\mu g$ per 100ml respectively. The output of these thyroid hormones from the thyroid is controlled by the thyrotropic hormone (TSH) produced in the pituitary gland.

Content in foods depends upon the concentration of iodide in the soil in which the plants grow. Analysis of foods for iodine is thus meaningless and no figures can be given. As a general guide fruits, vegetables, cereals and meats may contain up to $10\mu g$ iodine per 100g. A more realistic general figure is between 2 and $5\mu g$ per 100g. Seafoods provide the richest sources with amounts (in μg per 100g): haddock 659; whiting 65-361; herring 21-27.

Dried kelp is the richest source and contains from 0.535-6.87mg per g.

Excretion of iodine as iodides is mainly via the urine.

Functions of iodine reside solely in its presence in the thyroid hormones triiodothyronine and thyroxine. These hormones determine the level of metabolism in the body, i.e. the rate at which food is converted into energy and the way in which this energy is utilized. They also control the rate of growth in the growing child.

Deficiency of iodine is an important world health problem. At least 200 million people world-wide are estimated to be suffering from diseases related to deficiency of the trace mineral. Iodine intake consistently under 50µg per day induces deficiency diseases. Lack of iodine gives rise to goitre; hypothyroidism or underactive thyroid; cretinism. Lack of thyroid hormones gives rise to myxoedema.

Causes of deficiency include:

1. reduced dietary intake of iodides;
2. excessive intakes of anti-thyroid foods which contain substances that prevent uptake of iodine by the thyroid, e.g. brassica, cabbage, cassava, kale, ground-nuts, soya beans, turnips and the seeds of cabbage, mustard and rape;
3. medicinal drugs e.g. para-aminosalicylic acid (used to treat tuberculosis); sulphonylureas (oral anti-diabetes agents); perchlorates (used to treat thyrotoxicosis); thiocyanates (used to reduce high blood-pressure); resorcinol (used to treat acne and seborrhoea in an ointment form but some is absorbed into the blood); iodine in large doses (inhibits release of thyroid hormones).

Symptoms of deficiency include apathy, drowsiness, sensitivity to cold, lethargy; muscle weakness, increase in weight. All are due to a sluggish metabolism. Accumulation of mucinous material under the skin giving a coarseness to its texture.

Therapeutic and supplementary forms of iodine are ammonium iodide; calcium iodide; calcium iodobehenate; potassium iodide; potassium iodate; sodium iodide; iodized table salt; iodized poppy-seed oil (injectable and long-acting); kelp; sea salt. These supply only iodine. If the deficiency disease is due to an inability to make the hormones with adequate iodine present only the hormones can be used therapeutically.

Recommended dietary intakes as suggested by the USA authority Food and Nutrition Board, National Academy of Sciences - National Research Council (in µg per day): infants 0-0.5 year, 35; 0.5-1.0 year, 45; children 1-3 yrs, 60; 4-6 yrs, 80; 7-10 yrs, 110; males 11-14 yrs, 130; 15-18 yrs, 150;

19-22 yrs, 140; 23-50, 130; 51 yrs + , 110; females 11-14 yrs, 115; 15-18yrs, 115; 19-22 yrs, 100; 23-50 yrs, 100; 51 yrs + , 80; during pregnancy, 125; whilst breast-feeding, 150.

UK and WHO authorities make no recommendations but agree that the normal daily intake in the diet is about 200μg, which should satisfy most requirements.

Excessive intakes of iodine as iodides give effects that are complicated in nature. They include hyperthyroidism also known as thyrotoxicosis and Grave's disease; goitre and hypothyroidism in asthmatics on prolonged administration; increased relapse rate in those being treated with anti-thyroid drugs; myxoedema in those being treated with radioactive iodine for Grave's disease. Hyperthyroidism has been induced in those with goitre taking 180mg potassium iodide daily; in those with normal thyroid glands given iodine-containing drugs or radio-diagnostic contrast media containing iodine. Iodine worsens dermatitis herpetiformis in those with the disease and should be avoided by them.

The UK General Sales List restricts the daily dose of iodine to 10mg for non-prescription medicines. *See also* iodism.

---

iodine poisoning, symptoms of acute poisoning from ingestion of elemental iodine are mainly due to its corrosive effects on the gastrointestinal tract. It causes a disagreeable metallic taste; vomiting; abdominal pain and diarrhoea. Eventually the kidneys fail to produce urine, and swelling of the throat due to oedema or oedema of the lump follows. The fatal dose is 2 to 3g of elemental iodine. Maximum permissible atmospheric concentration is 0.1ppm. Large volumes of milk and starch solutions with 1 per cent solution of potassium thiosulphate are needed in emergency treatment of swallowed iodine.

---

iodism, hypersensitivity to iodine itself or more rarely iodides after prolonged oral administration. Symptoms are: a severe cold in the head (coryza); headache; pain in the salivary glands; watery eyes; weakness; conjunctivitis; fever; laryngitis; bronchitis; skin eruptions; skin rashes; exacerbation of acne.

---

iodized table salt, the addition of sodium or potassium iodide or potassium iodate to table salt to ensure no lack of iodine in the general population. It is carried out in the USA, Switzerland, Yugoslavia, New Zealand and some countries of South America. Salt is not iodized in the UK.

In the USA iodized salt must contain 76μg iodine per g salt. Daily consumption of table salt is estimated at between 2 and 6g providing 152-456μg iodine. New Zealand suggests 84.7μg iodine per g salt. Other countries recommend lower levels in table salt that appear to be just as effective. Salt used in the processing and refining of foods is not usually iodized.

---

iron,　chemical symbol Fe, from the Latin *ferrum*. Atomic weight 55.85. Second most abundant metal in earth's crust after aluminium. Occurs naturally as haematite, magnetite, limonite and siderite. Can exist in two forms known as ferrous and ferric iron.

Essential trace mineral constituent of the body being necessary for haemoglobin (the red pigment of blood) formation. Occurs also in oxidation enzymes (cytochromes) of living tissues. The body contains between 3.5 and 4.5 grams of iron of which two-thirds is present as haemoglobin, the remainder being stored as protein-iron complexes called ferritin and haemosiderin in the liver, spleen and bone-marrow. About 3 per cent is present as an iron-containing pigment called myoglobin in muscle cells where it acts as an oxygen reservoir within the muscle fibres. Less than 0.1 per cent of total body iron circulates in the blood plasma (i.e. the straw-coloured fluid in which the blood cells are suspended) where it is bound to a protein called transferrin.

In food iron is present in both organic and inorganic forms known respectively as haem and non-haem iron. Haem iron is associated with meat foods and is absorbed unchanged. Non-haem iron is found in other foods and must be reduced to the ferrous form before it can be absorbed. Hence ascorbic acid (vitamin C) is needed for optimum absorption of non-haem iron and iron in supplements since it ensures all iron is in the ferrous state and helps to carry it across the intestinal wall.

The level of *body iron stores* is a function of dietary intake and intestinal iron absorption. When body stores are low, the amount absorbed is increased. Only between 5 and 15 per cent of food iron is normally absorbed from a diet that supplies 15-20mg per day. Hence in a good diet from 6-16mg per day passes unabsorbed with the faeces. Absorption is greatest in childhood and tends to be reduced in later years.

About 0.6-1.0mg of body iron is excreted daily in sweat, bile, urine and faeces and lost in the nails, hair and the skin. As the amount absorbed from an ordinary diet is 1.0-1.5mg per day, most individuals are just in positive iron balance. When losses are additional under normal conditions such as menstruation (0.5-0.8mg per day) and lactation (0.4mg per day), deficiency can readily occur if such losses are not made up by higher intakes. Increased amounts of 25 per cent must be taken during pregnancy to cater for the demands of the foetus.

Iron enters into several *metabolic cycles* in the body. The predominant one involves haemoglobin synthesis where a total of 800-900g is made and destroyed about every 120 days. Most of the 21-24mg of iron released daily by this process is conserved by the body for re-synthesis into new haemoglobin. All absorbed iron is bound to the protein transferrin and transported to the bone-marrow where it is incorporated into haemoglobin of the red blood cells. Some iron is shunted to other storage sites in the liver and spleen and, to a lesser extent, other body cells. The quantity of iron that transferrin can bind normally ranges between 250 and 400mg per 100ml. Only 30-40 per cent of transferrin carries iron so normal plasma iron content ranges from 60-200mg per 100ml. Plasma iron content is usually reduced in chronic debilitating disease or infection. It is increased when red blood-cell destruction is excessive during diminished red blood-cell production or when there is abnormal release of body iron stores as in acute liver disease.

Iron absorption from the food is influenced by other food factors. In the absence of sufficient vitamin C, absorption of non-haem iron is impaired. A high intake of phytic acid found in raw cereals and raw vegetables will immobilize iron in the form of iron phytate that cannot be absorbed. Foods high in phosphates will prevent iron absorption by forming insoluble iron phosphate. The tannic acid of tea and other beverages reacts with iron resulting in production of non-absorbed iron phytate. Meat iron is unaffected by other food constituents and is the best absorbed form of the mineral.

High intakes of vegetable foods in a meal slightly reduce the absorption of meat iron. Meat in a meal doubles the amount of iron absorbed from maize and beans. None of the factors reducing non-haem iron absorption affect that of haem iron.

The percentage iron absorbed from various foods is: veal 20; liver 15; blood 13; fish 11; soya beans 8; lettuce 5; corn 4; beans 3; spinach 1.5; rice 1.0.

Iron deficiency is the most widespread mineral nutritional deficiency worldwide. In poorer countries it is due to high intakes of phytic acid-containing foods with little if any iron from meat, fish and dairy products.

Also in the Third-World countries many of the population suffer from intestinal worms and parasites that cause increased loss of blood from the gastrointestinal tract as well as taking iron from the food for their own use. In general, women in their child-bearing years are at greatest risk from iron deficiency because without an iron-rich diet they are unlikely to make up the blood lost in the menstrual flow during each monthly cycle. Deficiency too is likely in pregnancy and during breast-feeding if extra iron is not eaten. These extra demands on women's stores of iron are compensated by their greater ability to absorb the mineral than men. Deficiency can be a feature of both men and women who suffer regular bleeding from gastric and duodenal ulcers; from haemorrhoids (piles); as a side-effect of drugs like aspirin and other anti-arthritic remedies which cause gastric bleeding; from growths in the gastrointestinal tract; from losses of blood during operations; from excessive alcohol intake; from acholorhydria (lack of acid in stomach); low levels of vitamin C and the trace mineral copper in the diet can cause iron deficiency because both nutrients are needed to ensure efficient absorption of iron. Infants may be prone to iron deficiency when fed on cow's milk because its iron content is low. Hence dried cow's and goat's milks are usually fortified with the mineral. Placental transfer of iron is also not very efficient, so most of the baby's needs must be met from a milk source until weaning starts to contribute meaningful amounts.

The functions of iron include its presence in the red pigment of blood haemoglobin where it acts as an oxygen carrier; its presence in myoglobin, the oxygen reserve protein of muscles; its presence in intracellular enzymes known as cytochromes which function as oxygen carriers inside the body cells; its presence in catalase, an intracellular enzyme that destroys the toxic material hydrogen peroxide produced by some of the body's metabolic processes. There is a relationship between iron in the body cells and the resistance to disease. The mineral forms an essential part of the enzymes and immune substances necessary to destroy invading micro-organisms. An iron-containing enzyme called myeloperoxidase is essential for the production of the white blood cells which repel and destroy invading bacteria. Low body levels of iron reduce the capacity of the bone-marrow to produce white blood cells so anti-infective defences are weakened. Piglets when born are notoriously low in iron and are most susceptible to infection until body-iron levels build up. Similarly, people with low haemoglobin (from low iron) blood levels are more prone to respiratory infections and chronic infections of the teeth, gums, ears and skin. The lower the iron level in body tissues, the less the resistance to infective micro-organisms.

Increasing iron intake can reduce the chances of infection.

The signs of iron deficiency are in general related to the anaemia that results from low blood levels of haemoglobin and hence reduced oxygen-carrying capacity. They include in the early stages tiredness, fatigue and lack of stamina. There is pale complexion; pallor of the inside of the eyelids replacing the normally pink membrane, and lack of the usual red flare spreading from the half-moons of the fingernails. Later symptoms include breathlessness, giddiness, dim vision, headaches, insomnia, palpitation, fast pulse rate, heart murmers, loss of appetite, indigestion, tingling in the fingers and toes — all associated with decreased oxygen supplies to the tissues and organs.

The ultimate test is measurement of the blood haemoglobin level. In adults this should be within the range of 12-16g per 100cc of blood. Less than 12g per 100cc is considered to be anaemia and some 10 per cent of British women have haemoglobin at this level. One per cent have a haemoglobin of less than 8g per 100cc at which stage the heart output of blood may be affected. Iron-deficiency anaemia accounts for few deaths but it contributes greatly to the general unhealthy condition and substandard performance of millions of people.

Generalized itching (pruritus), particularly in later life, may occur around the arms, the legs, the genitals and the abdomen. It may be related to lack of iron in the blood plasma rather than in the red blood cells since anaemia is not always present. Increased iron intake will often help relieve the problem. In young children, iron deficiency results in depressed growth and impaired mental performance.

Therapy for iron deficiency includes increased intake of iron-rich foods in the diet; oral supplementation with iron preparations; intramuscular injection of iron complexes.

Foods rich in iron include (in mg per 100g): boiled cockles 26.0-40.0; dried yeast 20.0; cooked liver 7.5-17.0; cooked kidney 6.4-17.0; boiled winkles 15.0; wheat bran 12.9; cocoa powder 10.5; low-fat soya flour 9.1; parsley 8.0; full-fat soya flour 6.9; dried peaches 6.8; oysters 6.0; canned sardines 4.6; dried figs 4.2; dried apricots 4.1; oatmeal 4.1; boiled spinach 4.0; wholemeal flour 4.0; dried prunes 2.9; corned beef 2.9; wholemeal bread 2.5; boiled haricot beans 2.5; beef 1.9; sultanas 1.8; white bread 1.7; raisins 1.6.

Supplementary iron is presented as amino-acid chelated iron; ferrous aspartate, ferrous carbonate saccharated; ferrous citrate; ferrous fumarate; ferrous gluconate; ferrous iodide; ferrous orotate; ferrous succinate; ferrous sulphate, ferric acetate; ferric albuminate; ferric ammonium acetate; ferric ammonium citrate; ferric citrate; ferrice fructose; ferric glycerophosphate, ferric oxide saccharated, ferric phosphate; ferric pyrophosphate.

Iron salts added to white flour in breadmaking include: ferric ammonium citrate; ferrous sulphate; iron powder. Injectable preparations include iron-dextrin complex; iron-dextran complex; saccharated iron oxide; iron sorbitol.

Recommended daily intakes of iron in the UK are (in mg): 0-1 year, 6; 1-3 yrs, 7; 4-6 yrs, 9; 7-10 yrs 10; males 11-14 yrs, 12; 15-18 yrs, 12; 19-22 yrs, 10; 23-50 yrs, 10; 51 yrs and over, 10; females 11-14 yrs, 12; 15-18 yrs, 12; 19-22 yrs, 12; 23-50 yrs, 12; 51 yrs and over, 10. During pregnancy and lactation recommended daily intakes should be increased to 13 and 15mg respectively.

In the USA recommended intakes are higher (in mg): 0-1 year, 10; 1-3 yrs, 15; 4-6 yrs, 10; 7-10 yrs, 10; males 11-14 yrs, 18; 15-18 yrs 18; 19-22 yrs, 10; 19-22 yrs, 18; 23-50 yrs, 10; 51 yrs and over, 10. During pregnancy and lactation recommended intakes should be increased to 18mg daily.

Excessive iron intakes may lead to a disease called haemosiderosis, a generalized deposition of iron within body tissues, or haemochromatosis when such deposition is associated with tissue injury. Haemochromatosis is uncommon and is of a hereditary nature. Typical manifestations are cirrhosis of the liver; bronze pigmentation of the skin; diabetes mellitus; heart disease especially congestive failure, arrhythmias and conduction disturbances; loss of libido; abdominal pain; arthritis and liver cancer. Haemosiderosis can be caused by haemolytic anaemias; liver disease; massive blood transfusions; excessive iron injections, high oral intakes from food, wine, beer and cider prepared in iron utensils over many years.

Accidental poisoning with ferrous sulphate, usually in children, can be fatal. As little as 3g of this substance has caused death in a small child.

Side-effects noted with oral iron preparations include pain above the stomach, colic and constipation. Up to 20 per cent of persons taking iron may suffer.

---

iron amino-acid chelate, provides 10mg ferrous iron in 100mg. Daily supplementary dose is 24mg iron. Best absorbed and assimilated form of iron with less side-effects than conventional iron salts.

---

iron dextran injection, provides 50mg of iron in 1ml. Given by deep intramuscular injection. Toxic effects include pain, staining at the site of injection, and allergic reactions. Intravenous injection may cause headaches, nausea, vomiting, flushing, sweating and difficulty in breathing.

iron hydroxide, a food additive used as a brown colouring agent, E172. Also designated Colour Index Nos. 77472; 77499. Provides 62.2mg iron per 100mg. Acceptable daily intake up to 0.5mg per kg body weight. Permitted as a colouring agent in specified sugar products; in certain jam products.

iron oxide, a food additive used as yellow, red, brown or black colouring agent depending on composition; E172. Also designated Colour Index Nos. 77489; 77491; 77499. Mixture of three types of iron oxide providing from 70.0-77.8mg iron per 100mg. Acceptable daily intake up to 0.5mg per kg body weight. Permitted as a colouring agent in specified sugar products; in certain jam products.

iron phosphate, a mixture of ferrous phosphate, ferric phosphate and oxides of iron. Provides 16mg iron in 100mg plus 5.9mg phosphorus. Has advantage of being only slightly astringent. Daily dose is 0.3-2.0g.

iron sorbitol injection, provides 50mg iron in 1ml. Daily dose 1 or 2ml by deep intramuscular injection. Toxic effects may occur 30 minutes after injection and include metallic taste or loss of taste, flushing, nausea and vomiting. Occasionally dizziness, headache, joint pains, cardiac arrhythmias and low blood pressure occur. Allergic reactions are not uncommon.

Itai-itai, also known as 'ouch-ouch', a disease reported in Japan that is probably associated with high intakes of cadmium from eating rice grown on land irrigated with high cadmium-containing water. Characterized by kidney and gastro-intestinal lesions together with bone softening and severe bone pain similar to that in osteomalacia. Symptoms occurred mainly in older women, particularly those who had borne many children, and in those consuming diets low in protein, vitamin D and calcium. Cadmium may be antagonistic to dietary calcium causing severe deficiency of it.

itching, also known as pruritus. A generalized form is sometimes associated with old age. Blood plasma iron levels are usually low despite no iron-deficiency anaemia present. Condition apparently due to response of skin nerves to local iron deficiency. Treatment is with 60mg of elemental iron three times daily. Response is usual within a few days of therapy.

K

kelp, popular name for the seaweed ascophyllum nodosum. Also known as tangle and knotted wrack. Grows in abundance on the west-facing coasts of Europe which are exposed to the Gulf Stream. It feeds through its fronds (leaves) and is attached to rock by holdfasts. Minerals from sea water are concentrated in the body of the plant. After collection from the sea the plant is dried at temperatures between 75 and 85°C then ground to a fine powder. It may be added in this form to foods but is usually taken in the form of compressed tablets. Sometimes the powder is extracted with water and only the aqueous extract is used — the solids content of the extract is usually about 10 per cent.

Kelp is an excellent source of many minerals but it is usually taken for its iodine content. A typical analysis of kelp is (in mg per gram): potassium 19.8; sodium 16.4; calcium 12.3; nitrogen 12.1; sulphur 4.6; magnesium 2.5; phosphorus 1.0. Trace minerals present include (in μg per gram): iodine 535; iron 220; zinc 43; manganese 38; nickel 10; copper 4; cobalt 3; bromine, chromium, lead, strontium, vanadium, all 1; molybdenum 0.1.

Another species laminaria hyperborea is particularly rich in iodine, containing from 5.8-6.8mg per gram, i.e. some ten times more potent than kelp. *See also* kelpware.

kelpware, popular name for the dried thallus (filament without a root) of fucus vesiculosus, fucus serratus and fucus siliquosus. Also known as bladder-wrack, sea-wrack, bladder fucus, black-tang, cut-weed, sea-oak. Found in the Atlantic and Pacific oceans. Mineral contents are similar to those in kelp. *See* kelp.

Keshan disease, a congestive heart disease that is potentially fatal, affecting children and prevalent in vast areas of rural China. Clinical studies indicate that when given 1000μg selenium per week, affected children were cured of heart disease. When the selenium supplement was given to all members of a commune, incidence of the disease became zero.

---

kidney, rich in iron, zinc and copper, but poor source of calcium and magnesium. Both sodium and potassium are present in similar amounts and it is a good source of sulphur and phosphorus. For all varieties of kidney, range of mineral levels (in mg per 100g) are: sodium 180-400; potassium 180-340; calcium 8-16; magnesium 15-29; phosphorus 230-360; iron 5.0-12.0; copper 0.42-0.84; zinc 1.9-4.7; sulphur 170-290; chloride 180-520.

---

kidney stones, also known as renal calculi. Most are made up of insoluble calcium oxalate. The stones cause pain, fever, obstruction of the urinary tract, infection and blood in the urine. Evidence from clinical studies now suggests that such stones can be prevented by suppressing calcium levels with extra magnesium. Quantities required were 200-300mg elemental magnesium daily. Supplementary magnesium has been found to suppress kidney-stone formation in those prone to them; the mineral has also helped remove pre-formed stones in some cases. Vitamin B$_6$ supplementation may complement the action of magnesium since the vitamin is concerned in the mineral's metabolism.

L

---

lamb, good source of iron, zinc and copper. Some cuts are low in sodium but added salt increases intake. Useful potassium, phosphorus, chloride and sulphur levels but low in calcium and magnesium. All cuts when cooked, contain minerals in the following ranges (in mg per 100g): sodium 33-250; potassium 100-380; calcium 4-11; magnesium 10-28; phosphorus

100-240; iron 0.9-2.7; copper 0.08-0.33; zinc 1.4-6.9; sulphur 120-290; chloride 50-350.

---

laverbread, rich source of iron with good quantities of zinc and copper. High sodium and chloride food because of salt addition during making and good potassium content. Useful supplier of magnesium and phosphorus but poor calcium level. Made from edible seaweed, it contains the following minerals (in mg per 100g): sodium 560; potassium 220; calcium 20; magnesium 31; phosphorus 51; iron 3.5; copper 0.12; zinc 0.8; chloride 820.

---

lead, chemical symbol Pb from the Latin *plumbum*. Atomic weight 207.2. One of the metals known to the ancient world. Occurs in the earth's crust to the extent of 0.002 per cent, mainly as the mineral galena in which it is combined with sulphur.

Traces of lead appear to be essential for the health of some animals but never shown as a necessary trace mineral for man. Problem is one of excessive intakes rather than deficiency.

Excessive intakes may occur from food, drinking water and the air. Exhaust fumes from petrol-driven vehicles are the main source of atmospheric lead which has a maximum permissable concentration of 150μg per cubic metre. In Los Angeles air concentration was 4.5μg per cubic metre in 1969 which contributed significant extra intake. In the UK a survey of drinking water in 43 boroughs indicated that 96 per cent of the population in those boroughs consumed water with a pH less than 7.8 which was sufficiently acid to dissolve lead from piping. In soft-water areas lead piping can give rise to levels of 108μg lead per litre water. Main water supply was only 17.9μg per litre, indicating significant dissolution of lead. Food levels of lead reflect the extent of the metal in the water that irrigates the land on which the food is grown. Home-made beer and wine made in pewter vessels can also contribute significant amounts of lead by dissolution.

Total dietary intake of lead in industrialized societies is between 200 and 400μg daily. Ninety per cent of this is unabsorbed and excreted in the faeces; most of the remainder is got rid of through the kidneys. Some stays behind and a blood level above 42μg per 100ml is associated with lead poisoning.

Toxic effects are well documented in children who are more susceptible to lead poisoning than adults. Poisoning has come from accidental ingestion of lead salts; from lead toys and by sucking lead-painted articles. Acute poisoning causes intense thirst; metallic taste in the mouth; burning abdominal pain; vomiting; diarrhoea; black stools; lack of urine formation; shock; coma. Chronic poisoning is insidious, causing loss of appetite; constipation; headache; weakness; a blue or black lead-line on the gums; anaemia. Later there is vomiting; irritability; inco-ordination; neuritis leading to unsteady gait, visual disturbance, delirium; paralysis (with wrist and foot drop); kidney failure. Acute abdominal pain may result; in pregnancy the uterus violently contracts inducing abortion. Organic lead compounds like those in petrol-vehicle exhaust fumes have a specific action on nervous tissues. Mental disturbances are often a feature; and convulsions may occur.

Anaemia is often the first sign of lead intoxication but it is seldom severe and is characterized by large numbers of immature red blood cells.

---

leeks, low sodium food with high potassium levels. Good calcium and iron content but only small amounts of other minerals. In the raw and boiled states respectively, mineral levels (in mg per 100g) are: sodium 9, 6; potassium 310, 280; calcium 63, 61; magnesium 10, 13; phosphorus 43, 28; iron 1.1, 2.0; copper 0.10, 0.09; zinc 0.1, 0.1; sulphur 49, 49; chloride 43, 43.

---

leg ulcers, caused by a breakdown of healthy skin resulting from poor blood circulation; often a feature of deep vein thrombosis, varicose veins and diabetes. Have been treated successfully by a combination of oral zinc supplements (200mg three times daily) and directly applied zinc ointment containing zinc, silver (as silver nitrate) and allantoin (from comfrey) at the 1 per cent strength.

---

lemon curd, useful iron and zinc contents but low in most other minerals. Richest source of minerals is present in the home-made variety as opposed to the commercial starch-based product. Figures (in mg per 100g) for starch-based and home-made respectively, are: sodium 65, 150; potassium 11, 66; calcium 9, 18; magnesium 2, 5; phosphorus 15, 62; iron 0.5, 0.6; copper 0.03, 0.06; zinc 1.3, 0.4; sulphur 42, 48; chloride 150, 220.

---

lemonade, bottled variety supplies traces only of the minerals magnesium, potassium, iron and chloride. Low levels of the following (in mg per 100g): sodium 7, potassium 1; calcium 5; copper 0.01.

lemons, both fruit and juice are virtually sodium free, but supply good potassium levels. Small amounts only of other minerals. Figures for edible part and fresh juice respectively (in mg per 100g) are: sodium 6, 2; potassium 160, 140; calcium 110, 8; magnesium 12, 7; phosphorus 21, 10; iron 0.4, 0.1; copper 0.26, 0.13; zinc 0.1, trace; sulphur 12, 2; chloride 5, 3.

lentils, low sodium food rich in iron, copper and zinc trace minerals. Good source of potassium and magnesium with useful quantities of phosphorus and sulphur. In raw and boiled state respectively (in mg per 100g) mineral content is: sodium 36, 12; potassium 670, 210; calcium 39, 13; magnesium 77, 25; phosphorus 240, 77; iron 7.6, 2.4; copper 0.58, 0.19; zinc 3.1, 1.0; sulphur 120, 39; chloride 64, 20.

lettuce, low sodium food providing good potassium levels. Useful quantities of trace minerals. Mineral content is (in mg per 100g): sodium 9; potassium 240; calcium 23; magnesium 8; phosphorus 27, iron 0.9; copper 0.03; zinc 0.2; chloride 53.

lime juice cordial, small amounts of most minerals but potassium content is useful. In undiluted form it contains the following minerals (in mg per 100g): sodium 8; potassium 49; calcium 9; magnesium 4; phosphorus 5; iron 0.3; copper 0.07; chloride 4.

lithium, chemical symbol Li. Atomic weight 6.9. An alkali metal. Occurrence in earth's crust is 0.005 per cent by weight as the minerals spodumene, lepidolite, petalite and triphylite.

Lithium is not considered to be an essential trace mineral in animals or man but it is usually supplied to the body in drinking water. Studies on communities differing in lithium content of their drinking water suggest that higher intakes of the mineral result in lower death-rates from heart attacks; lower number of admissions for mental disorders; lower suicide rates; lower murder rates; lower incidence of gastric and duodenal ulcers; lower incidence of gout; lower incidence of rheumatism. Low lithium levels in water were found to be 8mg per litre; high levels were 100mg per litre. Some South American Indian communities known for their quiet, peaceful ways and reduced incidence of arthritic complaints, gastroduodenal ulcers and heart disease have been found to have lithium intakes from their drinking water some 50 times more than the average Western World community.

Absorption of lithium is very efficient and is passive, requiring no specific absorption process. It is rapidly distributed throughout the body with highest concentrations occurring in the bones, the thyroid gland and the brain. Most excretion occurs through the kidneys into the urine and there are also losses in the sweat and saliva. The mineral crosses the placenta in the pregnant female and also appears in the breast milk of the nursing mother. All information on distribution throughout the body has come from studies on people given high doses of lithium. It cannot be detected easily in the body when the sole source is dietary.

Food sources of lithium are not known as levels have not been measured. Concentrations in drinking water can range from 4-150mg per litre and this represents the main source for most people.

Functions of lithium include that of a mood stabilizer. This has been utilized in psychiatry where the mineral is given as a treatment for mania and in the prevention of manic depression and depression. It could also be acting in a similar manner in those communities who have a high intake from their water supply but the evidence is based only on epidemiological studies.

How it functions is unknown. Observed effects of lithium when given in drug doses are:

1. increased turnover of the hormone noradrenaline;
2. displacement of sodium from extracellular fluids;
3. reduction of bone mineral content;
4. increased blood serum concentrations of magnesium, calcium and phosphate;
5. increased blood plasma level of parathormone (from the parathyroid glands) which controls calcium and phosphorus metabolism;
6. a reduced synthesis and release of thyroid hormones;
7. an increased release of insulin enhancing formation of muscle glycogen;
8. increase in blood plasma level of anti-diuretic hormone (vasopressin);

9. transient increase in blood plasma level of aldosterone.

Therapy with lithium in acute mania requires constant monitoring of the plasma concentration to ensure that this lies close to 0.7mg per 100ml. At this level there is no interference with sodium and potassium levels. If lithium concentration rises above 1.4mg per 100ml adverse effects will appear. Treatment must therefore be left in the hands of a medical practitioner who has access to a blood plasma monitoring service.

In the past, lithium has also been used to treat leucopenia (low white blood cell count), hyperthyroidism, Ménière's disease, tardive dyskinesia, Huntington's chorea; and in the management of migraine, cluster headache, epilepsy, premenstrual syndrome. Many of these non-psychiatric uses are anecdotal and need to be investigated further. Doses of blood serum concentrations of lithium for use in these disorders have not been standardized.

Therapeutic forms of lithium are lithium carbonate; lithium citrate; lithium chloride; lithium sulphate; lithium aspartate; lithium gluconate; lithium orotate; lithium acetate. All are classed as prescription drugs only.

Excessive intakes give rise to nausea; vomiting; diarrhoea; coarse tremor; sluggishness; defective speech at blood plasma levels greater than 1.05mg per 100ml. At higher levels, i.e. greater than 1.4mg per 100ml the mineral gives rise to manifestations of impaired consciousness; abnormal muscle tenseness; coarse tremor; twitchings; increased reflex action; epileptic fits; 'coma vigil', where the individual can react when spoken to only by moving the head or eyes.

---

lithium acetate,   provides 10.2mg lithium in 100mg acetate.

---

lithium aspartate,   provides 9.4mg lithium in 100mg aspartate.

---

lithium carbonate,   provides 18.7mg lithium in 100mg carbonate.

---

lithium chloride,   provides 16.4mg lithium in 100mg chloride.

---

lithium citrate,   provides 7.3mg lithium in 100mg citrate.

---

lithium gluconate,   provides 3.4mg lithium in 100mg gluconate.

---

lithium orotate,   provides 4.4mg lithium in 100mg orotate.

---

lithium sulphate,   provides 10.8mg lithium in 100mg sulphate.

---

liver,   rich in potassium, phosphorus, sulphur and provides also sodium and chloride. Excellent source of the trace minerals iron, copper and zinc. Range of mineral quantities for all varieties (in mg per 100g): sodium 110-240; potassium 250-410; calcium 22-26; phosphorus 350-470; iron 7.5-17.0; copper 0.53-12.0; zinc 3.4-8.2; sulphur 250-300; chloride 120-250.

---

loganberries,   practically sodium free and providing good potassium and iron intakes. Useful quantities of other minerals present.

Figures for raw, stewed without sugar and stewed with sugar respectively (in mg per 100g) are: sodium, identical in all three states, 3; potassium 260, 240, 220; calcium 35, 32, 29; magnesium 25, 23, 21; phosphorus 24, 22, 20; iron 1.4, 1.3, 1.2; copper 0.14, 0.13, 1.2; sulphur 18, 17, 15; chloride 16, 15, 13.

Canned variety contains the following (in mg per 100g): sodium 1; potassium 97; calcium 18; magnesium 11; phosphorus 23; iron 1.4; copper 0.04; sulphur 3; chloride 5.

---

loss of taste,   also known as hypogeusia. A symptom associated with many conditions, e.g. head colds; pregnancy; old age. Associated also with copper deficiency; zinc deficiency; and vitamin deficiencies (especially vitamins A, B_6 and B_{12}). Loss of taste perception may be associated with a deficient protein in the saliva, known as gustin, that is a zinc-containing protein. Treating gustin-deficient people with zinc supplements (25mg of the element daily) restored gustin contents of the saliva to normal and the sense of taste returned. Studies have indicated that about one third of those with hypogeusia are zinc deficient. It is worth while, therefore, to take extra zinc as first-line treatment in any case of taste loss.

---

lychees, virtually sodium free with only small quantities of other minerals. Useful potassium level. In the raw and canned state respectively, mineral content is (in mg per 100g): sodium 3, 2; potassium 170, 75; calcium 8, 4; magnesium 10, 6; phosphorus 35, 12; iron 0.5, 0.7; copper 0, 0.11; zinc 0, 0.2; sulphur 19, 0; chloride 3, 5.

M

---

macaroni, pasta prepared from wheat flour. It is a low sodium food supplying reasonable amounts of potassium, phosphorus, iron and zinc. Other minerals are present in small amounts. Quantities for raw and boiled respectively (in mg per 100g) are: sodium 26, 8; potassium 220, 67; calcium 26, 8; magnesium 57, 18; phosphorus 150, 47; iron 1.4, 0.5; copper 0.07, 0.02; zinc 1.0, 0.3; sulphur 95, 29; chloride 31, 10.

---

magnesia, also known as magnesium hydroxide. Milk of magnesia is suspension of 7-8 per cent magnesium hydroxide in water containing 0.1 per cent citric acid and natural oils as flavouring agents. Name is a trademark in UK and some other countries. *See also* cream of magnesia.

---

magnesium, chemical symbol Mg. Atomic weight 24.31. An alkaline earth metal. Name is derived from the Greek city Magnesia where there are large deposits of magnesium carbonate. One of the most common elements of the earth's crust present to the extent of 2.1 per cent by weight. Found naturally as magnesite, carnallite, dolomite, epsomite, kieserite and many other minerals.

Fourth most plentiful metal in the body which contains about 25g. Fifty per cent is found in the bone in combination with phosphate and bicarbonate and is not readily exchangeable with extracellular fluid which contains only 1 per cent of body magnesium. One-fifth of body mineral is present in the soft tissues mainly bound to protein. Blood plasma levels are normally between 1.4 and 2.4mg per 100ml and these are maintained largely by dietary intake combined with kidney and intestinal conservation. If dietary intake falls, the body conserves magnesium by excreting less in the intestine and kidneys.

Foods rich in magnesium are (in mg per 100g): soy beans 310; cashews 267; almonds 252; Brazil nuts 225; peanuts 167; dried brewer's yeast 231; wholewheat flour 140; brown rice 119; dried peas 116; shrimps 110; wholemeal bread 93; rye flour 92. Good sources are seafoods 40 to 90; bananas 42; dried fruits 60-80; meats 25-50; and vegetables 20-60.

Chlorophyll, the green pigment of plants and vegetables, provides 2.7g magnesium in 100g, but chlorophyll itself is present only to the extent of 0.1 per cent in fresh greens. One pound of greens thus supplies only 12mg magnesium in the form of chlorophyll but a total of 95mg of the element.

Cereals and vegetables represent the main sources of magnesium in normal diet, providing more than two-thirds of the daily intake.

Functions of magnesium are:

1. as cofactor in many enzyme systems including the energy-producing processes involving phosphate transfer; DNA replication; energy pumps maintaining correct distribution of sodium, potassium and calcium across cell membranes;
2. as essential cofactor in vitamin B_1 functioning;
3. as essential cofactor in vitamin B_6 functioning;
4. as stabilizer of the internal structure of the body cells with calcium and proteins by forming a bridge to stiffen all-membrane structure;
5. in growth of the body;
6. in repair and maintenance of body cells and tissues as cofactor in protein metabolism;
7. as cofactor in hormones;
8. as component of chlorophyll, essential in plants for the conversion of light energy into chemical energy — a process on which all life ultimately depends;
9. as an intracellular mineral essential for nerve impulse transmission.

Causes of deficiency include:

1. reduced dietary intake as in poor diet, malnutrition, anorexia nervosa, high raw bran intake, loss of appetite;
2. high dietary intakes of phosphorus, calcium, vitamin D and fats;
3. reduced or impaired absorption caused by malabsorption conditions; chronic diarrhoea induced by laxative abuse, gastrointestinal infections or allergies;

4. excessive urinary losses induced by kidney disease; by diabetes; by acute and chronic alcoholism; by cancer; by increased parathyroid hormone production; by vitamin D intoxication; by synthetic drug diuretics; by certain antibiotics, e.g. gentamycin; by anti-cancer drugs; by heart drugs such as digoxin; by increased aldosterone hormone production; by aldosterone hormone therapy; by increased thyroid hormone production; by thyroxine therapy; by low potassium intakes or depletion of potassium by increased excretion; by increased phosphate excretion; by muscle-wasting diseases;

5. excessive losses of other body fluids induced by prolonged sweating; by increased breast-milk output; by prolonged suction of nasal and gastric fluids during clinical and operative procedures; by gastrointestinal fistulae; by burns;

6. metabolic disturbances associated with parathyroid gland removal (hungry bone syndrome); with uncontrolled re-feeding after starvation; with intravenous feeding of glucose and amino acids; with insulin treatment of diabetes; with treatment of acidosis in kidney failure; with stressful situations like pain, major surgery, shock and worry; with acute pancreatitis; with high refined carbohydrates diets including excessive sugar intakes; with cirrhosis of the liver; with congestive heart failure; with nephrotic syndrome;

7. gastrointestinal losses caused by diarrhoea and malabsorption (see (3) above); by enteritis; by colitis; by short-bowel syndrome produced surgically; by enemas;

8. prolonged intravenous therapy without magnesium supplementation;

9. prolonged use of the contraceptive pill;

10. allergy to cow's milk in babies and infants;

11. high intake of milk in diet — milk has low magnesium-phosphorus ratio which restricts absorption of magnesium.

Deficiency symptoms in animals include nerve-muscle over-excitability; inco-ordination; behavioural alterations; seizures; tetany; irregular heartbeats. Severe deficiency in animals leads to inflammation of the blood vessels; thrombosis of the heart, main blood vessels, liver, brain and kidney; atherosclerosis; high blood pressure. *In man* they include loss of appetite; nausea; apathy; weakness; tiredness; vertigo; epilepsy and convulsions; nervousness; anxiety; muscle cramps; muscle tremors; tongue jerks and tremors; contraction of the facial muscles induced by a light tapping of the facial nerve (Chvostek's sign); nystagmus — rapid involuntary movements of the eye up and down or from side to side; ataxia — shaky movements and unsteady gait; insomnia; hyperactivity in children;

constipation; rapid heartbeat; irregular heartbeat; palpitations; enhanced digitoxin toxicity; hypoglycaemia — low blood sugar; oesophageal (gullet) spasms; painful swallowing (dysphagia); abnormal ECG tracings.

Therapy with magnesium has been used in treating premenstrual tension, a condition associated with low red blood cell magnesium; menstrual cramps; toxaemia of pregnancy; eclampsia, where at the end of pregnancy or shortly after childbirth the woman develops wholesale convulsions and passes into a coma; morning sickness in pregnancy; hypoglycaemia or low blood sugar; atherosclerosis, arteriosclerosis; heart condition such as angina, abnormal and irregular heartbeats; digitoxin toxicity and overdose; some cancer conditions; prolonged diuretic drug usage; epilepsy; alcoholism; loss of magnesium in diabetics; retinopathy due to diabetes; kidney stones consisting of calcium oxalate; chronic constipation due to spasm in intestinal sphincters or lack of contractility of the digestive system; hyperactivity in children; behavioural disorders in children; insomnia; mental depression, muscle cramps; excessive caffeine intake; epilepsy; deficiency in mother due to breast-feeding; chronic diarrhoea; other deficiency symptoms mentioned above.

Heart disease relationship to low body magnesium levels is suggested by epidemiological studies and animal evidence. Death-rates from coronary artery disease and from sudden arrhythmias are higher in areas of the world where water supplies are soft than where they are hard. Most critical mineral missing in soft water is magnesium. In soft-water areas, accident victims have significantly lower heart-muscle magnesium levels than do accident victims in hard-water areas. Those who die from ischaemic (lack of blood supply to muscle) heart disease have even lower levels of magnesium in the heart muscle. This suggests that high magnesium levels of hard water confer some protection against heart disease.

Where death-rate from heart and blood vessels diseases is highest the calcium-magnesium ratio in the diet is also high. In Finland and the United States, this ratio is high and so is cardiovascular disease mortality. In Japan where the ratio is low, mortality from cardiovascular disease is also low. High ratio is due to magnesium lack rather than calcium excess.

Animal studies indicate that low magnesium intake increases heart disease and that increased magnesium intakes are protective against heart disease. Animals fed diets similar to those eaten in affluent countries by most of the population caused spontaneous heart attacks in 80 per cent of experimental animals. These diets are high in fats (which prevent magnesium absorption), cholesterol, vitamin D, sodium, phosphate and protein but low in magnesium and potassium. Increasing magnesium intakes to five times the daily requirements reduced drastically all heart-disease manifestations.

Therapy of heart disease with magnesium has been reported to be beneficial in patients with acute and chronic heart disease, including angina. The mineral was used successfully in arrhythmias when given intravenously in acute cases. Congestive heart failure itself depletes magnesium levels as do diuretics and the drug digitalis, so therapy with the mineral is necessary to replace serious losses. Magnesium also depresses conduction and abolishes abnormal impulse formation so this explains some of its therapeutic effects. Magnesium depletion reverses these effects. Concurrent administration of potassium with magnesium is probably more beneficial.

Recommended dietary intakes of magnesium are those of the Food and Nutrition Board of the National Academy of Science — National Research Council in the USA. WHO and UK bodies make no recommendations since these authorities assume that everyone's diet is replete in the mineral. USA authorities recommend the following daily requirements (in mg); Infants 0-0.5 year, 50; 0.5-1.0 year, 70; children 1-3 yrs, 150; 4-6 yrs, 200; 7-10 yrs, 250; males 11-14 yrs, 350; 15-18 yrs, 400; 19 yrs and on, 350; females 11-14 yrs, 300; 15 yrs and on, 300; during pregnancy, 450; during lactation, 450.

Supplementary forms are magnesium amino-acid chelate; dolomite (present as magnesium carbonate); magnesium acetate; magnesium carbonate; magnesium chloride; magnesium citrate; magnesium gluconate; magnesium orotate; magnesium oxide; magnesium sulphate.

Toxic effects of magnesium are flushing of the skin, thirst, low blood pressure, loss of reflexes and respiratory depression. Excessively high blood levels lead to anaesthesia and eventually heart failure. Toxicity is common only in those with kidney failure given magnesium supplement or drugs containing the mineral. Above toxic effects have not been reported in other individuals taking supplements but excess magnesium may act as a purgative by irritating the bowel.

Treatment of severe magnesium intoxication is a purely medical matter involving circulatory and respiratory support combined with intravenous administration of calcium gluconate.

---

magnesium acetate,   provides 11.2mg in 100mg acetate. Used as a source of magnesium in solutions for kidney dialysis.

---

magnesium amino-acid chelate,   provides 10 or 18mg magnesium in

100mg chelate. Daily supplement is up to 1.67g chelate (providing 300mg magnesium at higher level). Claimed to be the best absorbed form of magnesium.

magnesium carbonate, provides the magnesium source of dolomite. Contains 25.2mg magnesium per 100mg carbonate. Used mainly as a weak antacid and mild laxative but in the form of dolomite is taken as a supplement. As an antacid dose is 250-500mg repeated according to needs; as a laxative dose is 2-5g.

Also used as a food additive. Functions as an alkali; as anti-caking agent. Acceptable daily intake is not limited. Permitted in certain cocoa products; in table salt; as a miscellaneous additive.

magnesium chloride, provides 11.8mg magnesium in 100mg chloride. Used intravenously and in solutions for kidney dialysis as well as orally. Dose is 8-30g daily providing between 944mg and 2400mg magnesium but higher level is that for mild purgative use.

magnesium citrate, provides 16.2mg magnesium in 100mg citrate. Presented as a sweet, effervescent solution. Main use is as a mild purgative.

magnesium gluconate, provides 5.3mg magnesium in 100mg gluconate. Daily dose is from 3-6g providing 158-316mg magnesium. Used also as 10 per cent solution in muscular and intravenous injections.

magnesium glycerophosphate, provides 12.5mg magnesium and 15.9mg phosphorus in 100mg glycerophosphate. Dose is usually 300-600mg up to a daily intake of 4g. Used mainly as a tonic.

magnesium hydroxide, constituent of milk of magnesia used only as an antacid (dose 500-750mg repeated as necessary) and as a laxative (dose 2-4g daily).

Also used as a food additive. Functions as an alkali. Acceptable daily intake not limited. Provides 41.4mg magnesium per 100mg. Permitted in certain cocoa products; as a miscellaneous additive.

magnesium orotate, provides 6.9mg magnesium in 100mg orotate. Synthetic derivative alleged to be better absorbed than magnesium salts.

magnesium oxide, presented as heavy and light types that vary only in density. Both provide 59.5mg magnesium in 100mg oxide. As an antacid, dose is 250-500mg (providing 149-298mg magnesium) as needed but supplementary intake is 500mg oxide daily. As a laxative dose is 2-5g daily.

Also used as a food additive. Functions as alkali; anti-caking agent. Acceptable daily intake not limited. Permitted in certain cocoa products; as a miscellaneous additive.

magnesium phosphate, used only as an antacid and mild laxative but largely replaced by magnesium trisilicate. Usual dose is 1-4g repeated as necessary. Provides 20.4mg magnesium plus 17.6mg phosphorus in 100mg.

magnesium stearate, consists of a mixture of magnesium stearate and magnesium palmitate, prepared from magnesium and vegetable oils (or sometimes animal fats). Used in dusting powders in skin diseases and in cosmetics. Acts as mechanical barrier in barrier cream. Added to tablets as a lubricant to prevent tablets sticking during manufacture but quantity used is usually only up to 5mg per tablet.

Provides about 4.5mg magnesium in 100mg stearate so when used as lubricant adds only 0.2mg magnesium to tablet. Not used as a supplement because of its water insolubility. Inhalation of magnesium stearate by babies can cause toxic effects but no evidence that small amounts used as tablet lubricant are harmful.

Used also as a food additive. Functions as an emulsifier; an anti-caking agent; a release agent. Acceptable daily intake not limited. Permitted as a miscellaneous additive.

magnesium sulphate, also known as Epsom Salts. It is a common ingredient of aperient mineral waters. Rarely used as a supplement although when taken for its mild purgative effect significant amounts may be absorbed. Should not be taken by those with impaired kidney function and by children with intestinal parasitic diseases. Acts in dilute solution when swallowed by reducing the normal absorption of water from the intestine with the result that the bulky fluid contents distend the bowel and evacuation of the contents of the intestine follows in 1 or 2 hours.

Provides 9.7mg magnesium in 100mg sulphate. As a purgative dose is 5-15g sulphate in 250ml water, preferably before breakfast. For children dose is 100-250mg sulphate per kg body weight.

Used also as a food additive. Functions as a dietary supplement; as a firming agent; in brewing. Acceptable daily intake has not been determined. Permitted in boiler feed water for direct steam treatment of milk; as a miscellaneous additive.

---

magnesium trisilicate, used only as an antacid (0.5-2.0g repeated as necessary) when it exerts its effect slowly. Prolonged action is of value in the management of gastric and duodenal ulcers.

Also used as a food additive. Functions as an anti-caking agent. Acceptable daily intake not limited. Provides 18.5mg magnesium and 32.3mg silicon per 100mg. Permitted miscellaneous additive.

---

mandarin oranges, low sodium food with useful amounts of potassium, iron and zinc. *Canned variety* contain the following levels of minerals (in mg per 100g): sodium 9; potassium 88; calcium 18; magnesium 9; phosphorus 12; iron 0.4; copper 0.05; zinc 0.4; chloride 2.

---

manganese, chemical symbol Mn. Atomic weight 54.9; occurs in the minerals pyrolusite, hausmannite, manganite, manganosite, brannite. Present in minute quantities in water, plants and animals. Widely distributed in the earth's crust at an abundance of 0.085 per cent. An essential trace element for human beings.

The body of an adult person contains between 12 and 20mg. Highest concentrations are found in the skeleton, liver, kidneys and heart. Excretion of manganese is via the bile so most is lost in the faeces. Daily losses are usually about 4mg. Only from 3-5 per cent of dietary manganese is absorbed so daily intakes must be sufficient to allow for these losses.

Food sources are (in mg per 100g): oat flakes 4.94; wholemeal bread 4.28; wheatgerm 4.2; avocados 4.2; chestnuts 3.7; hazel nuts 3.48; rye bread

3.07; peas 1.99; almonds 1.94; coconut 1.31; olives 1.2; pineapple 1.07; rice 1.01; plums 1.0; spinach 0.83; lettuce 0.78; white bread 0.71; bananas 0.64; blackberries 0.59; beetroot 0.58; watercress 0.54; calf liver 0.34; Brazil nuts 0.32; beef liver 0.3; oysters 0.295; carrots 0.25; honey 0.21; asparagus 0.19; potatoes 0.17; cauliflower 0.17; peaches 0.11; cabbage 0.11; apples 0.08; eggs 0.033; oranges 0.025; mackerel 0.02; haddock 0.015; halibut 0.01; pork 0.01; cow's milk 0.002.

Functions of manganese include:

1. the control of growth at all stages of development;
2. maintenance of a healthy nervous system;
3. presence as an essential cofactor in many enzyme systems including those concerned with active phosphate transfer and production in the synthesis of bone cartilage;
4. presence in female hormones;
5. presence as an essential cofactor in the production of nucleic acids, the basic building blocks of cells, that are also in the genetic code;
6. a role in thyroid hormone synthesis;
7. presence in enzymes required for the utilization of the B vitamins, vitamin C and vitamin E;
8. the synthesis of glycoproteins — combined sugars and proteins — that surround and protect every body cell;
9. the synthesis of interferon, the natural anti-viral and perhaps anti-cancer agent of the body;
10. the development and maintenance of healthy bones;
11. stimulation of glycogen (animal starch) formation in the liver.

Deficiency is usually related to poor dietary intake. Processing and refining of foods cause serious manganese losses. It may also be associated with copper excess.

Deficiency signs in animals include bone deformities; poor growth; shaky movements and unsteady gait in the newborn induced by inefficient calcium deposition in the inner ear (otoliths); lack of maternal instinct by a mother for her offspring. No specific deficiency signs have been reported in human beings.

Deficiency in human beings has been noted in diabetes; heart disease; schizophrenia; atherosclerosis; myasthenia gravis (weakness of the muscles); rheumatoid arthritis; infants before weaning.

Therapy has been found beneficial in schizophrenia; myasthenia gravis; anaemia — when it is alleged that manganese increases the efficacy of iron.

Supplementary forms of manganese are amino-acid chelate; manganese sulphate; manganese gluconate; manganese orotate; manganese chloride;

manganese glycerophosphate; manganese hypophosphite.

Recommended dietary intakes suggested by the WHO are 2.5mg daily for adults. Human diets provide from 1-8mg daily; the average British diet has been calculated to provide 4.6mg per day. Unrefined vegetarian diets contain more. Tea can provide up to half the daily intake in the tea-drinking countries like Australia and the UK. Authorities in the USA suggest the following daily intakes (in mg): infants 0-0.5 year, 0.5-0.7; 0.5-1 year, 0.7-1.0; children 1-3 yrs, 1.0-1.5; 4-6 yrs, 1.5-2.0; 7-10 yrs, 2.0-3.0; 11+ yrs, 2.5-5.0; adults, 2.5-5.0. These figures are recorded as both adequate and safe.

Excessive intakes of manganese from oral ingestion are rare. Symptoms include lethargy; involuntary movements; impairment of voluntary movement; changes in muscle tone; postural changes; coma.

Chronic poisoning from inhalation of manganese dust is an industrial hazard. Symptoms include irritation and infections of the respiratory system; headache; sleep disturbances; dermatitis; irritability; liver enlargement; nerve degeneration similar to Parkinson's disease. Other symptoms include weakness in the legs; hand tremor; slurred speech; muscular cramps; fixed facial expression; mental deterioration; gastrointestinal irritation; excessive perspiration; excessive salivation; sexual disturbances; blood diseases. Maximum permissible atmospheric concentration is 5mg per cubic metre.

---

manganese amino-acid chelate, provides 10mg manganese in 100mg chelate. Alleged to be the best absorbed manganese supplement available. Usual dose is up to 100mg chelate daily.

---

manganese chloride, provides 27.7mg manganese and 35.9mg chloride in 100mg. Used in a similar manner as manganese sulphate. Daily dose in human beings is 25-100mg chloride.

---

manganese gluconate, provides 11.4mg manganese in 100mg gluconate. Used as a dietary supplement in animal feeds and in human beings. Daily dose in human beings is 100-200mg gluconate.

---

manganese glycerophosphate, provides 24.4mg manganese and

13.8mg phosphorus in 100mg glycerophosphate. Also known as manganese glycerylphosphate. Has been given in doses of 60-300mg daily in the treatment of debilitated conditions and in convalescence.

---

manganese hypophosphite, provides 27.1mg manganese and 30.6mg phosphorus in 100mg hypophosphite. Has been given in doses of 60-300mg daily in the treatment of debilitated conditions and in convalescence.

---

manganese orotate, provides 35.2mg manganese in 100mg orotate. Used as a dietary supplement in human beings. Daily dose is 25-75mg orotate.

---

manganese sulphate, provides 24.6mg manganese in 100mg sulphate. Has been added to ferrous sulphate in doses of 0.5-2.5mg manganese sulphate to improve iron utilization. Widely used in veterinary medicine to prevent or treat manganese deficiency. Usual human dose is 25-100mg sulphate daily.

---

mangoes, virtually sodium free with good quantities of potassium. Some trace minerals present. Mineral levels for raw and canned variety respectively (in mg per 100g) are: sodium 7, 3; potassium 190, 100; calcium 10, 10; magnesium 18, 7; phosphorus 13, 10; iron 0.5, 0.4; copper 0.12, 0.09; zinc 0, 0.3; chloride 0, 5.

---

marmalade, low sodium and potassium levels but supplies useful quantities of calcium and iron. Levels of the following minerals (in mg per 100g) are: sodium 18; potassium 44; calcium 35; magnesium 4; phosphorus 13; iron 0.6; copper 0.12; sulphur 2; chloride 7.

---

marrow, sodium free with good potassium content. Small amounts of trace minerals present. Mineral levels supplied by raw and boiled respectively (in mg per 100g) are: sodium 1, 1; potassium 210, 84; calcium 17, 14; magnesium 12, 7; phosphorus 20, 13; iron 0.2, 0.2; copper 0.03, 0.03; zinc 0.2, 0.2; sulphur 0, 6; chloride 30, 14.

---

marzipan, excellent source of potassium and is also low in sodium. Rich source of calcium, magnesium and phosphorus. Good source of iron, zinc and sulphur. Mineral levels are (in mg per 100g): sodium 13; potassium 400; calcium 120; magnesium 120; phosphorus 220; iron 2.0; copper 0.08; zinc 1.5; sulphur 81; chloride 13.

---

melons, all types are low in sodium and supply very good levels of potassium. Some trace minerals present.

Canteloupe variety, levels for raw, edible portion (in mg per 100g): sodium 14; potassium 320; calcium 19; magnesium 20; phosphorus 30; iron 0.8; copper 0.04; zinc 0.1; sulphur 12; chloride 44.

Honeydew variety, levels for raw, edible portion (in mg per 100g): sodium 20; potassium 220; calcium 14; magnesium 13; phosphorus 9; iron 0.2; copper 0.04; zinc 0.1; sulphur 6; chloride 45.

Watermelon, raw, edible portion, contains the following levels (in mg per 100g): sodium 4; potassium 120; calcium 5; magnesium 11; phosphorus 8; iron 0.3; copper 0.03; zinc 0.1.

Menke's syndrome, is a rare genetic disease characterized by an inability of the baby to absorb copper, resulting in progressive degeneration of the nervous system. Deterioration starts with convulsions at three months of age and death used to occur within three years. Symptoms and signs are failure to keratinize hair which looks like steel wool, hence the name 'steely-hair syndrome'; mental retardation; low body temperature; low copper levels in blood plasma and in liver; weakened skeleton; degenerative changes in the walls of the aorta. Provided diagnosis is made early in life, the condition can be controlled with intravenous copper.

---

menstrual cramps, abdominal cramps that tend to occur a few days before menstruation and may continue through the first few days of the menstrual flow. Has been found to respond, along with associated leg and back cramps, to supplementary calcium, 500-1000mg in the few days preceding menstruation until it has finished.

---

mercury, Chemical symbol Hg, from the Latin *hydrargyrum*. Atomic weight 200.6. Also known as quicksilver, liquid silver. Occurs in nature as cinnabar (mercuric sulphide) with an abundance in the earth's crust of 0.5mg per kg.

Not known to have any essential role in the metabolism of any living organism. In the form of liquid or gaseous mercury it is toxic. Mercury salts and particularly organic forms of mercury are more poisonous than the element. Dental amalgams used for filling teeth cavities are so insoluble that they are usually not regarded as toxic but some doubts expressed recently on the safety of the tiny amounts eroded from fillings. Claims that cancer, heart disease, menstrual and thyroid problems relieved by removal of amalgam fillings. The most dangerous forms of mercury are the alkyl derivatives methylmercury and ethylmercury. They are usually introduced into the body from fish and grain foods.

Inorganic mercury salts, introduced by pollution into fresh and sea waters, are converted by micro-organisms into methylmercury. This is introduced into the food chain via plant-eating small fish to carnivorous large fish like tuna, swordfish and pike. When these fish are eaten by man, poisoning results. Fatal levels of contamination in such fish have been reported from Japan where industrial pollution introduced mercury salts into sea water.

Fish from inland fresh-water lakes in Sweden and North America may contain as much as 503μg mercury per 100g which is a toxic level. Canned tuna can contain from 10-80μg mercury per 100g, half as methylmercury. Deep-sea fish caught off the UK fishing grounds contain only 8μg mercury per 100g, but nearer the coasts where chemical effluents are discharged into the sea, fish may contain up to 50μg mercury per 100g. The highest tolerable weekly intake of mercury according to WHO recommendations is 300μg, of which no more than 200μg should be methylmercury.

Seeds that have been dusted with alkyl mercury compounds to prevent fungal contamination have caused poisoning in Guatamala, Iraq and Pakistan. The poisoning was accidental since the seeds were not meant for human consumption but 459 deaths resulted from 6500 cases. Similar treated seeds fed to farm animals have given rise to mercury poisoning in humans who ate the meat from these animals.

Elemental mercury may arise from accidental breaking of thermometers, barometers; from discarded batteries, mercury vapour lamps, mercury switches; from coal burning, which can contribute 3000 metric tons per year to the atmosphere; from natural weathering of rocks and soils which contribute 230 metric tons annually; from the 'silvering' of coins; from manufacture of mercury amalgams.

Ingested mercury compounds accumulate in certain parts of the brain, eventually causing brain damage. Other affected organs include the colon and kidneys. Methylmercury causes nerve degeneration; birth defects; genetic defects; chromosome damage; excessive salivation; loss of teeth; gross muscle tremors. When applied to the skin, alkyl mercury compounds cause irritation, redness and blistering.

In babies, dusting of the skin with powders or application of ointments containing mercury causes pink disease or acrodynia. Characterized by lesions of the skin on the hands and feet; swelling of the extremities; digestive disturbances; itching of the hands and feet; pink coloration of hands, feet, cheeks and tip of nose; weakness of the muscles; arthritis.

Acute poisoning by soluble mercury compounds causes metallic taste; thirst; severe abdominal pain; vomiting; ashy discoloration of the mouth and throat; diarrhoea contaminated with blood. Later ulceration, kidney disease and colitis with severe haemorrhage may develop. Mercury vapour when inhaled causes respiratory symptoms and kidney damage.

Chronic poisoning by mercury vapour or by soluble mercury salts or by prolonged skin contact causes tremor; muscle instability; sensory disturbances; gastrointestinal symptoms; dermatitis; liver and kidney damage; anaemia; mental deterioration. A blue line on the gums may be indicative of chronic mercury poisoning.

Maximum permissible atmospheric concentrations of mercury are $50\mu g$ per cubic metre air and $10\mu g$ alkyl mercury per cubic metre of air.

Medicinal compounds of mercury include:
1. ammoniated mercury to treat impetigo and threadworm infections;
2. oleated mercury, as ammoniated mercury;
3. mercurial diuretics, used in cardiac oedema;
4. mercuric chloride, used in solution as a disinfectant for the skin;
5. mercuric cyanide, used as a disinfectant in eye solutions;
6. red mercuric iodide, used as a disinfectant in wounds; as a vaginal douche; as a skin disinfectant; to treat ringworm and lupus; to treat syphilis;
7. mercuric nitrate, used to treat syphilitic warts; eczema; psoriasis;
8. yellow mercuric oxide, used as an ointment to treat blepharitis; conjunctivitis. Prolonged use should be avoided as mercury can be absorbed through eye tissues.
9. Mercuric oxycyanide, preferred over mercuric chloride as a skin disinfectant and in eye lotions;
10. mercurous chloride, once used orally as a purgative, dose 30-200mg, but now discontinued because of absorption. As an ointment or dusting powder has been used to treat itching; psoriasis and eczema; as a strong ointment (30-50 per cent) in preventing syphilis.

migraine, a particular type of headache caused by constriction of the head blood vessels followed by their dilation which gives rise to pulsating pain. Extra magnesium taken at the rate of 400mg daily, preferably as the amino-acid chelate, has been claimed to prevent development of migraine headaches. A trigger factor for the development of those headaches may be high concentrations of sodium in some sufferers. One study has shown that those people could precipitate migraine attacks by sudden loads of common salt as in potato crisps, salted nuts, and high sodium foods such as pickles, sauces and preserved meats; or of sodium glutamate in highly spiced and oriental foods. Avoiding these foods led to a reduced incidence of migraines in these people.

---

milk, liquid forms are fairly low in sodium but contain good levels of potassium. Very rich source of calcium with useful quantities of all other minerals. Dried variety is richer in all minerals (including sodium) because of concentration effect.

Cow's milk, fresh, whole contains the following mineral levels (in mg per 100g): sodium 50; potassium 150; calcium 120; magnesium 12; phosphorus 95; iron 0.05; copper 0.02; zinc 0.35; sulphur 30; chloride 95.

Sterilized, levels (in mg per 100g): sodium 50; potassium 140; calcium 120; magnesium 12; phosphorus 95; iron 0.05; copper 0.02; zinc 0.35; sulphur 30; chloride 100.

Fresh, skimmed milk supplies the following (in mg per 100g): sodium 52; potassium 150; calcium 130; magnesium 12; phosphorus 100; iron 0.05; copper 0.02; zinc 0.36; sulphur 31; chloride 100.

Dried, skimmed milk supplies (in mg per 100g): sodium 550; potassium 1650; calcium 1190; magnesium 117; phosphorus 950; iron 0.40; copper 0.20; zinc 4.1; sulphur 320; chloride 1100.

Goat's milk contains (in mg per 100g): sodium 40; potassium 180; calcium 130; magnesium 20; phosphorus 110; iron 0.04; copper 0.05; zinc 0.30; chloride 130.

Human milk, mature supplies the following (in mg per 100g): sodium 14; potassium 58; calcium 34; magnesium 3; phosphorus 14; iron 0.07; copper 0.04; zinc 0.28; chloride 42.

---

milk of magnesia, *see* magnesia.

---

mincemeat,   good source of potassium but added salt increases sodium level. Provides good intakes of iron and copper. Contains the following mineral levels (in mg per 100g): sodium 140; potassium 190; calcium 30; magnesium 10; phosphorus 17; iron 1.5; copper 0.20; zinc 0.2; chloride 200.

---

mineral absorption,   the process whereby minerals are transferred from the food or from supplements into the intestinal cells and hence into the bloodstream. The main site of absorption of minerals is the small intestine but some are transferred in other parts of the gastro-intestinal tract. Simple minerals like sodium, potassium, chloride and iodide that are present as electrically charged atoms (known as ions) are absorbed by simple diffusion from the gut contents into the intestinal cells and there is little or no control of their absorption. Control of their level in the body comes in their excretion. Sodium, potassium, lithium and ammonium ions are monovalent, i.e. they carry only one positive charge. They cannot be chelated for this reason. Calcium, magnesium, copper, zinc, iron and manganese are all divalent, i.e. they carry two positive charges per atom. Small amounts of them may also be assimilated by simple diffusion, but in the main they must be chelated with amino acids before they can be absorbed into the intestinal cells and hence into the bloodstream. Transport of divalent minerals within the body is mainly as complexes with amino acids or with proteins but small amounts exist in the bloodstream as simple ions, e.g. calcium, which participates in the blood-clotting process. Absorption of divalent minerals therefore depends upon:

1.   the quantity of protein or amino acids present in the digestive system;
2.   the quality of protein or amino acids available, since the right sort of amino acids must be present;
3.   competition amongst minerals for the amino acids available and the specific sites of absorption in the small intestine. For example, lead and iron compete for the same sites; cadmium and zinc compete for the same sites. Any excess of one mineral over its competitor will increase its chances of absorption.

Table 5 shows the ratios of quantities of minerals absorbed from amino-acid chelates compared with these from mineral salts and oxides.

Table 5: The ratios of quantities of minerals absorbed from amino-acid chelates compared with those from mineral salts and oxides

Mineral	Amino-acid chelates: Carbonates	Amino-acid chelates: Sulphates	Amino-acid chelates: Oxides
Copper	5.8:1	4.1:1	3.0:1
Magnesium	1.8:1	2.6:1	4.2:1
Iron	3.6:1	3.8:1	4.9:1
Zinc	3.0:1	2.3:1	3.9:1

mineral content of vegetables, in general the mineral content of vegetables reflects that of the soil in which they are growing. Studies have indicated that even in plants growing in adjacent areas, there is wide variation in mineral content because of differing soil concentrations. Other factors may also play a part — see minerals in soil. Table 6 illustrates how vegetables may not always contain the concentrations of minerals expected. However it must be pointed out that most mineral concentrations in vegetables sold commercially lie somewhere in the middle of the ranges.

Table 6: Variation in mineral content of selected vegetables

Food	Figures in p.p.m. (parts per million)	Boron	Manganese	Iron	Copper	Cobalt
Snap beans	Highest content	73	60	227	69	0.26
	Lowest content	10	2	10	3	0.00
Cabbage	Highest content	42	13	94	48	0.15
	Lowest content	7	2	20	0.4	0.00
Lettuce	Highest content	37	169	516	60	0.19
	Lowest content	6	1	9	3	0.00
Tomatoes	Highest content	36	68	1938	53	0.63
	Lowest content	5	1	1	0	0.00
Spinach	Highest content	88	117	1584	32	0.25
	Lowest content	12	1	19	0.5	0.20

mineral losses in freezing, are made up of leaching of minerals during the thawing process; losses into water during the blanching stage; losses into the water or fat during the cooking processes. Typical losses of calcium and magnesium from frozen fruits and vegetables are shown in Table 7.

Table 7: Typical percentage losses of calcium and magnesium from frozen fruits and vegetables

Fruits and vegetables	Calcium	Magnesium
Apricots	33	12
Asparagus	0	30
Blackberries	56	48
Black-eyed peas	7	0
Blueberries	53	0
Brussels sprouts	33	9
Cherries	22	0
Corn	57	53
Green beans	19	34
Green peas	4	31
Lima beans	33	28
Peaches	33	40
Potatoes	0	38
Spinach	0	23
Strawberries	39	31

mineral losses in refining, all minerals are lost to some extent during the refining of natural foods into the processed variety, but losses of trace minerals are the most significant. Some of these are shown in Table 8.

Table 8: Percentage losses of trace elements by refining of foods

	Co	Cr	Cu	Fe	Mg	Mn	Mo	Se	Zn
White flour from wholemeal	89	98	68	76	85	86	48	16	78
Polished rice from brown rice	38	75	25	—	83	27	—	—	50
White sugar from raw cane sugar	88	90	80	99	99	89	—	75	98
Refined oils from cold expressed oils	—	—	—	—	99	—	—	—	75
Butter production from milk	—	—	—	—	94	—	—	—	50

Gross minerals too are lost (see Table 9). In the UK and some other countries calcium and iron must be replaced at levels of between 94 and 156mg calcium and not less than 1.65mg iron per 100g flour in white flour, but there is no legislation regarding all other minerals.

Table 9: Percentage losses of gross minerals by refining of wheat and sugar

	Ca	Cl	K	Na	P	S
White flour from wholemeal	60	0	77	78	71	32
White sugar from raw cane sugar	96	99	98	99	99	99

mineral relationships, the minerals in the body are all in balance with one another so that excess or otherwise of one or more will affect the levels of others. Their relationships are summed up in the mineral wheel shown in Figure 1.

Figure 1: Mineral relationships

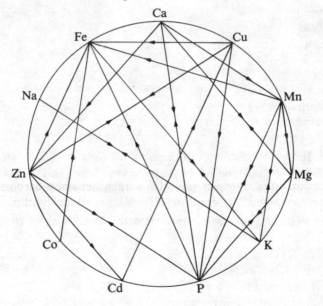

Ca - Calcium, Cd - Cadmium, Co - Cobalt, Cu - Copper,
Fe - Iron, K - Potassium, Mg - Magnesium, Mn - Manganese,
Na - Sodium, P - Phosphorus, Zn - Zinc

On this wheel an arrow pointing to a particular mineral means that a deficiency of that mineral may be caused by an excess of the mineral from whence the arrow comes. For example, a high calcium intake may reduce the amount of zinc; high cadmium intakes will cause copper levels to drop. When the line between two minerals contains two opposing arrows, each mineral may influence the other. A low potassium intake will allow sodium to accumulate and conversely an excess of sodium in the diet will lower potassium levels in the body.

The wheel allows other relationships to be worked out. Calcium and/or phosphorus deficiency may allow an excess of manganese to develop. This high level can cause depression of potassium which allows sodium to accumulate. There is no direct line between calcium and sodium and potassium but calcium levels can indirectly affect those of the other two elements. Hence calcium deficiency may have an effect upon blood pressure. In another example calcium and/or phosphorus in excess will depress zinc levels leading to a skin disease called parakeratosis. This complaint can therefore be caused by excessive intakes of calcium and phosphorus as well as a reduced dietary intake of zinc.

---

mineral waters, have now been officially defined under EEC regulations. 'Natural mineral water' means water which originates in an underground water table or deposit and is extracted for human consumption from the ground through a spring, well, or other exit. 'Natural mineral water fortified with gas from the spring' means an effervescent mineral water whose carbon dioxide content includes carbon dioxide from the same water table or deposit as the water. 'Naturally carbonated mineral water' means an effervescent natural mineral water whose carbon dioxide content is the same after decanting (if it is decanted) and bottling as it was at source. It includes a natural mineral water to which carbon dioxide from the same water table or deposit as the water has been added if the amount added does not exceed the amount previously released during decanting or bottling. The only treatments allowed for natural mineral water are filtration or decanting; total or partial removal of carbon dioxide by physical methods; the addition of carbon dioxide only to mineral waters that are naturally effervescent. Hence chlorination, fluoridation and softening of natural mineral waters are not allowed.

Natural mineral waters vary widely in their content of minerals. A low mineral content water must not contain more than 500mg of mineral salts per litre. A very low mineral content water must not contain more than 50mg of mineral salts per litre. A water rich in mineral salts must contain more than 1500mg of mineral salts per litre. The following descriptions can only be used where the claimed mineral has a content in mg per litre above that stated: contains bicarbonate (600); contains sulphate (200); contains chloride (200); contains calcium (150); contains magnesium (50); contains fluoride (1.0); contains iron (1.0); contains sodium (200). An acidic mineral water must contain more than 250mg free carbon dioxide per litre. A mineral water suitable for a low-sodium diet must contain less than 20mg sodium per litre.

The upper limits on trace mineral contents (both essential and toxic) of natural mineral waters are (in μg per litre): arsenic (50); cadmium (5.0); cyanides (50); chromium (50); mercury (1.0); nickel (50); antimony (10); selenium (10); lead (10). No limits are suggested for nitrates and nitrites but in view of the undesirability of high intakes of these, they should be absent or present only in low concentration in natural mineral waters.

Mineral waters when sold in bottles or drunk at source as at spas have been popular for centuries as a remedy for various complaints, particularly those of the rheumatic kind. With modern knowledge that such diseases may be associated with mineral imbalance there would appear to be some logic in increasing mineral intakes for their diuretic, laxative and replacement effects. Many people prefer mineral waters because the water has not been softened, chlorinated, fluoridated and has had the minimum of pipe feeding before they drink it.

---

minerals in soil, man derives his food from plants or from animals that have eaten plants or from fish that have eaten plants. All plants whether growing on land or in water must derive their minerals from the soil or the sea. These sources are the ultimate source of all minerals. The richness of a soil as well as depending on the macro-elements nitrogen, phosphorus and potassium must also have present other less abundant but just as essential trace minerals. Deficiency of macro-elements does exist. Some lands are low in phosphate, hence the importance of the natural phosphate-rich fertilizer guano. Potassium is lacking in some areas and deficiency is made up by treating the land with potassium, often obtained from rich inland lakes like the Dead Sea. Nitrogen is usually supplied in the form of nitrates. Zinc deficiency is not unknown and it reflects in the health of the farm animals who live off plants grown on the soil. Supplementation of animal feeds with zinc is more usual than treating the soil.

Mineral deficiencies in the soil can produce disease in localized areas. Lack of iodine in the soil causes goitre. Magnesium deficiency of the soil in certain areas of France has been associated with a particular type of cancer. Some regions in Poland had a high incidence of leukaemia. The causative agents were found to be toxins produced by the soil micro-organism aspergillus flavus. This fungus flourishes in soil that is deficient in iron, copper and magnesium and has excessive concentrations of silicon and potassium. When this imbalance was corrected by correct fertilization of the soil (extra trace elements plus dolomite to supply calcium and magnesium) the fungus was controlled and the incidence of leukaemia dropped. Low levels of manganese and chromium in the soil appear from epidemiological studies to increase the chances of heart disease and atherosclerosis in those living in the area. In South Africa, molybdenum, copper and iron deficiencies in the soil have led to oesophageal cancer.

Mineral excesses of a toxic element in the soil can also produce disease. In Japan, faulty treatment of waste water from a mine led to pollution of a river with cadmium. The mineral was deposited in the soil from which the plants absorbed it. When the rice was eaten, the local population accumulated cadmium in the body and, combined with a low calcium and vitamin D intake, a concentration was reached that resulted in a bone disease that caused excruciating pain. *See* Itai-itai disease. Adjustment of the diet to give the correct balance of the essential minerals cured the complaint. In the Netherlands, some areas of high silicon content in the soil had a high incidence of all types of cancer that was reduced by treating the soil with calcium. This inhibited the uptake of silicon by plants. Excessively high soil concentrations of zinc and chromium have been associated with gastrointestinal cancer in some parts of the world. In India a raised water table made the topsoil in one area more alkaline. This increased the uptake of molybdenum and fluoride by sorghum plants (the staple diet). These uptakes led to copper deficiency. The result was that the population eating these plants were copper deficient but had excessive intakes of molybdenum and fluoride. The result was a crippling bone disease called genu valgum which was only remedied by balancing the intake of the essential minerals.

Uptake from the soil can be affected by:
1. high levels of humic acid which can bind minerals, making them unavailable;
2. the presence of other minerals, e.g., low levels of potassium or high levels of phosphate will render iron insoluble;
3. pH. This is a measure of acidity or alkalinity of the soil. From pH 0-6 is acid, from pH 8-14 is alkaline; pH 7 is neutral. At neutral pH most minerals are fully available to the plant. In highly acid soils only potassium, iron, manganese, copper and zinc can be absorbed. In highly alkaline soils phosphorus, potassium, sulphur and boron are freely available for

absorption. *See also* Mulder's chart.

---

molybdenum, chemical symbol Mo. Atomic weight 95.9. Occurs in nature as molybdenite and wolfenite with an abundance in the earth's crust of 1-1.5mg per kg. Essential in soil and in plants for its function in the processes for 'fixing' or utilizing nitrogen. Essential trace element for animals and man.

Its presence in plants depends upon the type of soil in which they are growing. Molybdenum is high in plants grown on neutral or alkaline soils with a high content of organic matter; it is low in those grown on acid, sandy soils. High molybdenum fertilizers encourage clover growth.

The total adult body content is 9mg, but its distribution is unknown apart from the liver which contains 0.29-0.48mg per 100g. Blood vessels vary within the range 0.3-6.7μg per 100ml. This wide variation reflects dietary intake.

Absorption from the diet is fairly efficient at a level of 50 per cent. Excretion is mainly in the urine.

Food sources are widespread and values are (in μg per 100g): buckwheat 485; lima beans 400; canned beans 350; wheatgerm 200; liver 200; soy beans 182; barley 138; lentils 120; oats 114; sunflower seeds 103; kidney 75; heart 75; green beans 66; whole wheat 60; yams 59; macaroni 51; maize 50; rye 50; eggs 50; cocoa 50; noodles 45; rice 47; chicken 40; wholemeal bread 26; spinach 26; potatoes 25; coconut 25; white bread 21; shellfish 20; melons 16; apricots 14; milk powder 14; raisins 11; watercress 10; butter 10; strawberries 9; cornflakes 8; carrots 8; tea 8; plums 6; cheese 5; fish 4; endives 4; banana 3; milk 3; celery 2; lettuce 2. Alcoholic beverages are useful sources of molybdenum: Scotch whisky contains 17μg per 100ml, beer contains 6μg per 100ml, wine contains 5μg per 100ml.

Functions of molybdenum include nitrogen fixation in soil and plants; prevention of dental caries; its presence in the enzyme xanthine oxidase which is responsible for iron metabolism and production of uric acid, itself an excretion product of nucleic acid breakdown; maintenance of normal sexual functions in the male.

Deficiency is associated solely with reduced dietary intakes, as in relying upon foods grown in molybdenum-deficient soils; large reliance on processed and refined foods from which the mineral is lost.

Deficiency signs in human beings are irritability; irregular heartbeat; lack of production of uric acid; coma.

Diseases associated with deficiency include dental caries; sexual impotence in men; cancer of the oesophagus (gullet).

Therapy may be expected to be beneficial in diseases associated with deficiency but no trials have been carried out. Molybdenum has been used to detoxify excess copper intakes.

Supplementary forms are potassium molybdate; sodium molybdate.

Recommended dietary intakes suggested by the Food and Nutrition Board, National Research Council — National Academy of Sciences of the USA are (in μg per day): infants 0-0.5 year, 30-60; 0.5-1.0 year, 40-80; children and adolescents 1-3 yrs, 50-100; 4-6 yrs, 60-150; 7-10 yrs, 100-300; 11 + yrs, 150-500; adults, 150-500. These figures are regarded as both adequate and safe.

Excessive intakes of molybdenum have been reported as causing:
1. gout (at intakes of 10-15mg per day) in areas of molybdenum-rich soil. High blood levels of uric acid are produced in the affected individuals.
2. increased urinary excretion of copper, producing deficiency of this trace mineral. High intakes of molybdenum from foods grown in molybdenum-rich soils were to blame.

Molybdenum toxicity from inhalation or from supplementation is unknown. In animals excessive intakes cause copper deficiency characterized by loss of hair colour.

---

monosodium glutamate,   also known as MSG; sodium hydrogen L-glutamate. A food additive that functions as a flavour enhancer. Acceptable daily intake up to 120mg per kg body weight — not to be given to infants under 12 weeks old. Provides 12.3mg sodium per 100mg. Permitted miscellaneous additive. Prohibited in foods specially made for babies and young children. *See also* Chinese restaurant syndrome.

---

mouth ulcers,   also known as canker sores; aphthous ulcers; aphthous stomatitis. Acute painful ulcers on the moveable oral mucosal lining, occurring singly or in groups. Reports of successful prevention of mouth ulcers by taking oral zinc supplement equivalent to 20-25mg element daily. Existing ulcers may respond to directly applied zinc creams, preferably with the mineral as zinc gluconate or mouthwashes containing zinc.

---

mulberries,   good source of iron and potassium and is virtually free of sodium. Provides the following quantities of minerals (in mg per 100g):

sodium 2; potassium 260; calcium 36; magnesium 15; phosphorus 48; iron 1.6; copper 0.06; sulphur 9; chloride 4.

Mulder's chart, in soil a complicated mixture of minerals is presented to a plant. The uptake of a particular mineral is under the influence of other minerals which can either stimulate or antagonize the absorption of that mineral. Zinc absorption by a plant is dependent upon phosphorus, iron and calcium. High phosphorus levels antagonize the uptake of zinc, copper and potassium; they also stimulate the uptake of magnesium. Interrelationships are shown in the Figure 2.

Figure 2: Plant uptake of minerals

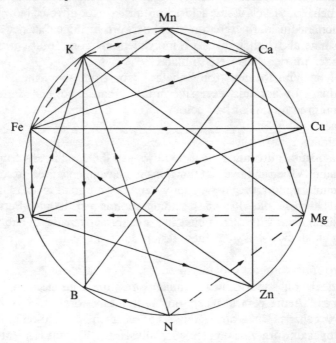

B - Boron, Ca - Calcium,
Cu - Copper, Fe - Iron,
K - Potassium, Mg - Magnesium,
Mn - Manganese, N - Nitrogen,
P - Phosphorus, Zn - Zinc.

———▶ Antagonism

— ▶ Stimulation

---

mung beans, low sodium food that is excellent source of iron, copper, potassium, calcium, magnesium and sulphur. In the raw state it supplies the following minerals (in mg per 100g): sodium 28; potassium 850; calcium 100; magnesium 170; phosphorus 330; iron 8.0; copper 0.97; sulphur 190; chloride 12.

---

muscle cramps, prolonged painful contractions of a muscle. May appear as spasms where the muscles cannot perform a specific task but allows the use of them for other movement. Known as occupational cramp, an example of which is 'writer's cramp'. Can be caused by an imbalance of certain minerals; also as a result of stress, bad posture or fatigue. May respond to extra calcium in the diet, usually between 640 and 800mg of the element daily. This therapy has been found to relieve 'growing pains' in children; night cramps; aching legs; muscle cramps of pregnancy. Night cramps may also respond to extra potassium in the diet. *See* fatigue.

---

muscular tics, also known as tremors and twitches. Repeated and largely involuntary movements of muscles varying in complexity. May become prominent under conditions of emotional stress. Caused by an impulse conductance abnormality at the junction of nerve and muscle, possibly due to a mineral imbalance. Most likely deficiencies are in potassium and magnesium. Supplementation with these minerals can often relieve persistent tics, tremors and twitches. May also be caused by excess toxic minerals like lead, in which case the condition is relieved by removal of the toxic mineral with agents calcium, zinc and vitamin C.

---

mushrooms, almost sodium free but rich in potassium. Supply good quantities of phosphorus, iron, copper and chloride. Mineral quantities for raw and fried respectively (in mg per 100g) are: sodium 9, 11; potassium 470, 570; calcium 3, 4; magnesium 13, 16; phosphorus 140, 170; iron 1.0, 1.3; copper 0.64, 0.78; zinc 0.1, 0.1; sulphur 34, 74; chloride 85, 100.

---

mustard and cress, low sodium food rich in potassium. Useful supplier of calcium, magnesium, phosphorus and sulphur and of the trace elements iron and copper. Contains the following mineral quantities (in mg per 100g): sodium 19; potassium 340; calcium 66; magnesium 27; phosphorus 66;

iron 1.0; copper 0.12; sulphur 170; chloride 89.

---

myxoedema, also known as hypothyroidism. The condition is caused by thyroid hormone deficiency in the adult. Symptoms and signs may be subtle and insidious at onset. The facial expression is dull; there is puffiness and swelling around the eyes; eyelids droop; hair is sparse, coarse and dry; skin is coarse, scaly, dry and thick; memory is poor; there is intellectual impairment with gradual change in personality; sometimes this leads to frank psychosis commonly called 'myxoedema madness'. Often carotene is deposited in the palms and soles causing yellow coloration. The tongue may be enlarged. Heartbeat rate is slow and the heart is often enlarged. Tingling in the hands and feet is often present. Reflexes are quick to contract but slow to relax. There may be excessive bleeding at menstrual periods. Constipation, low body temperature and anaemia are often present. Vitamin B_{12} absorption is adversely affected because of decreased intrinsic factor synthesis.

Treatment is replacement therapy with a variety of thyroid hormone preparations including synthetic thyroxine; synthetic triiodothyronine; combinations of both; desiccated animal thyroid. Average maintenance dose of 150-200µg L-thyroxine daily is the preferred treatment. At least 60 per cent of this is absorbed. In infants and young children maintenance dose is 2.5µg per kg body weight per day. Triiodothyronine tends to be used to initiate therapy because it has a rapid action and turnover, but this detracts from its use in long-term therapy where thyroxine is preferred.

Iodides cannot be used since the thyroid does not have the ability to convert them to the thyroid hormones. *See also* cretinism.

N

---

nectarines, virtually sodium free, supplying good potassium and iron levels. Mineral levels for the raw, edible portion (in mg per 100g) are: sodium 9; potassium 270; calcium 4; magnesium 13; phosphorus 24; iron 0.5; copper 0.06; zinc 0.1; sulphur 10; chloride 5.

---

nickel, chemical symbol Ni. Atomic weight 58.7. Occurs in nature as chalcopyrite, penthandite, garnierite, nicollite, nillerite; abundance in earth's crust 180mg per kg. It is an essential trace mineral for rats, chicks and swine, but functions not known.

Deficiency in animals impairs iron absorption leading to low iron levels in the tissues and organs and to iron-deficiency anaemia.

Not known to be essential for man but traces of the mineral are found in all human tissues.

Functions in animals include an antagonistic action to the hormone adrenalin; intensifying the action of insulin; increasing blood fats; stabilizing RNA and DNA in the tissues.

High blood levels are found in those who have suffered a heart attack; those with serious burns; those who have suffered a stroke; women with toxaemia of pregnancy; women with cancer of the uterus; those with lung cancer.

Low blood levels are found in those with cirrhosis of the liver; those with chronic kidney failure.

Food sources are provided by contamination, e.g. from the alloys used to line cooking utensils; from machines used to process and refine food, from pasteurization equipment; from margarine, where it is used as a catalyst in its production; from cigarette smoke. In tobacco some nickel combines with carbon monoxide to form the toxic nickel carbonyl, a known carcinogen (cancer-producing substance) for rats.

Toxic effects of excess oral nickel intakes in man are unknown. Nickel carbonyl from tobacco smoke may be a factor in causing lung cancer in man. Acute toxic effects of nickel carbonyl are frontal headache; vertigo; nausea; vomiting; chest pain; cough. Nickel when in contact with the skin of sensitive people can cause dermatitis.

Excessive oral intakes in young chicks cause pigmentation changes in the skin; swelling in the legs; dermatitis; fat-depleted liver; oxygen-depleted liver. The mineral accumulated in liver, bone and aorta.

O

---

oatmeal, low sodium food rich in potassium, magnesium, sulphur and phosphorus. Excellent source of trace minerals iron, zinc and copper. As raw, it gives the following mineral levels (in mg per 100g): sodium 33; potassium 370; calcium 55; magnesium 110; phosphorus 380; iron 4.1; copper 0.23; zinc 3.0; sulphur 160; chloride 73.

okra, practically devoid of sodium, it supplies good levels of potassium, calcium, magnesium and phosphorus. Useful quantities of trace minerals iron and copper. In raw state it supplies the following minerals (in mg per 100g): sodium 7; potassium 190; calcium 70; magnesium 60; phosphorus 60; iron 1.0; copper 0.19; sulphur 30; chloride 41.

olives, very high in sodium because of added salt. Supplies useful quantities of potassium and calcium with the trace minerals iron and copper. Olives in brine contain the following mineral levels (in mg per 100g): sodium 2250, potassium 91; calcium 61; magnesium 22; phosphorus 17; iron 1.0; copper 0.23; sulphur 36; chloride 3750.

onions, low sodium food providing good levels of potassium and sulphur. Spring variety is a good source of calcium, iron and copper. Mineral levels for raw and boiled respectively (in mg per 100g) are: sodium 10, 7; potassium 140, 78; calcium 31, 24; magnesium 8,5; phosphorus 30, 16; iron 0.3, 0.3; copper 0.08, 0.07; zinc 0.1, 0.1; sulphur 51, 24; chloride 20, 5.

As fried (in mg per 100g): sodium 20; potassium 270; calcium 61; magnesium 15; phosphorus 59; iron 0.6; copper 0.16; zinc 0.1; sulphur 88; chloride 38.

Raw, spring variety contains (in mg per 100g): sodium 13, potassium 230; calcium 140; magnesium 11; phosphorus 24; iron 1.2; copper 0.13; sulphur 50; chloride 36.

orange juice, similar mineral pattern to fruit — regarded as good source of potassium and some trace minerals. Fresh juice contains (in mg per 100g): sodium 2; potassium 180; calcium 12; magnesium 12; phosphorus 22; iron 0.3; copper 0.05; zinc 0.2; sulphur 5; chloride 1.

oranges, should be regarded as a low sodium food providing mainly high intakes of potassium. Useful quantities of trace minerals. The raw, edible portion supplies the following minerals (in mg per 100g): sodium 3; potassium 200; calcium 41; magnesium 13; phosphorus 24; iron 0.3; copper 0.07; zinc 0.2; sulphur 9; chloride 3.

---

orotates, synthetic complex of minerals with orotic acid. Some evidence that orotates are absorbed more efficiently than mineral salts from the intestine and they may act as carriers of certain minerals across cell membranes. Orotic acid has been named vitamin B_{13} in the past but as ample quantities are produced within the body as an intermediate in nucleic acid metabolism it is no longer regarded as a vitamin. Mineral orotates have been claimed to be beneficial in many clinical conditions. They are useful in replacing mineral deficiencies but some of the benefits in other conditions may be related to the orotic acid moiety.

---

osteoporosis, a honeycombing of the bones due to a decrease in bone tissue mass. Caused by a loss of calcium from the bone that is not replaced by normal resorption. The bones most commonly affected are the spinal vertebrae, the femur (thigh bone) and the radius (shorter arm bone). The condition is associated with the menopausal and post-menopausal female; prolonged use of oral corticosteriod drugs; excessive excretion of calcium on some medicinal drug treatments; overproduction of adrenal cortex steroid hormones; multiple myeloma; gastrectomy; prolonged immobilization. Dietary causes include insufficient intake of calcium over long periods; non-replacement of lost calcium in poorly-fed women with multiple births over many years; non-replacement of calcium lost in breast-feeding; increased effect of fluoride on copper deficiency, inducing osteoporosis of the legs; increased overnight loss of calcium after the menopause; increased urinary loss of calcium on high-protein diets. Symptoms may be absent until bone fracture occurs. Sometimes there is aching pain in the bones, particularly the back. X-ray analysis and biochemical measurements of the blood and urine are essential for correct diagnosis and to differentiate the condition from osteomalacia.

During the menopause and post-menopausal periods, medical treatment of osteoporosis is confined to hormone replacement therapy (HRT) with female sex hormones. This therapy is still being assessed for possible long-term, serious side-effects. Dietary treatment involves supplementation with calcium; with calcium and vitamin D to help absorb the calcium; sometimes with added fluoride to stimulate calcium resorption into the bones. Typical supplementary regimes are: 1000-1500mg calcium daily, preferably with 400IU vitamin D; 1000-1500mg calcium daily with 400 IU vitamin D plus 45mg per day sodium fluoride. In view of the toxicity of sodium fluoride, this regime should be taken only under medical supervision. Regular exercise is also an important factor in preventing and in treating osteoporosis. Adequate intake of calcium during life before the menopause also contributes to prevention of the disease once the menopause starts.

A decreased mineral density in the lumbar vertebrae of female athletes who have a reduced number of menstrual periods has been observed. Similar findings were noted in young women whose periods had stopped for reasons other than pregnancy. In all cases, calcium intake was suggested to be increased, from 800-1500mg per day.

P

Paget's disease,   also called osteitis deformans. A chronic degenerative disease of the bones occurring in the elderly and most frequently affecting the skull, backbone, pelvis and long bones. In the early stages of the disease calcium is lost from the bones. Characterized by deep, dull, aching bone pain that can cause headache, deafness, blindness when the skull is affected; bowing of the legs when these limbs are affected. Usual medical treatment is prolonged course of the hormone calcitonin but this may be complemented by extra calcium. Supplementary treatment consists of 500-1000mg calcium three times daily between meals, preferably in a form that does not supply phosphorus. Bone pain was relieved by this treatment which is believed to stimulate the body's own production of calcitonin.

papaya,   also known as pawpaw. Useful source of potassium, without sodium, and provides some trace minerals. When canned, contains the following minerals (in mg per 100g): sodium 8; potassium 110; calcium 23; magnesium 8; phosphorus 6; iron 0.4; copper 0.10; zinc 0.3; chloride 40.

parathyroid hormone, also known as parathormone. A polypeptide hormone containing 84 amino acids, synthesized in the parathyroid glands (adjacent to or embedded in the thyroid gland), that controls the distribution of calcium and phosphate in the body. Secretion of the hormone is stimulated by a decrease in blood calcium. A high concentration of the hormone causes transfer of calcium from the bone reservoirs to the blood; a deficiency lowers blood calcium levels, causing tetany. Hormone also functions by promoting formation of the active form of vitamin D within the kidney. This is probably how the hormone mediates in its action of increasing the absorption of calcium from the intestine. The hormone also decreases the kidney reabsorption of phosphate, allowing the mineral to be excreted.

parsley, very rich source of potassium and is low in sodium. Excellent supplier of calcium and iron. Useful quantities of phosphorus, copper and zinc. In raw state, it supplies the following mineral levels (in mg per 100g): sodium 33; potassium 1080; calcium 330; magnesium 52; phosphorus 130; iron 8.0; copper 0.52; zinc 0.9; chloride 160.

passion fruit, low sodium food, high in potassium and supplying useful quantities of magnesium, phosphorus and iron. As raw, it supplies the following mineral levels (in mg per 100g): sodium 28; potassium 350; calcium 16; magnesium 39; phosphorus 54; iron 1.1; copper 0.12; sulphur 19; chloride 37.

peaches, almost devoid of sodium but rich in potassium. Excellent source of iron, copper and zinc in the dried variety with good quantities of phosphorus and sulphur. As fresh, raw it contains these minerals (in mg per 100g): sodium 3; potassium 260; calcium 5; magnesium 8; phosphorus 19; iron 0.4; copper 0.05; zinc 0.1; sulphur 6; chloride trace.

Dried variety (in mg per 100g), as raw, stewed without sugar and stewed with sugar respectively: sodium 6, 2, 2; potassium 1100, 410, 390; calcium 36, 13, 13; magnesium 54, 20, 19; phosphorus 120, 44, 43; iron 6.8, 2.5, 2.4; copper 0.63, 0.23, 0.22; sulphur 240, 89, 85; chloride 11, 4, 4.

Canned peaches contain (in mg per 100g): sodium 1; potassium 150; calcium 4; magnesium 6; phosphorus 10; iron 0.4; copper 0.06; sulphur 1; chloride 4.

peanut butter, excellent source of potassium, magnesium, phosphorus and chloride; also the trace minerals iron, copper and zinc. High in sodium because of added salt. It supplies the following minerals (in mg per 100g): sodium 350; potassium 700; calcium 37; magnesium 180; phosphorus 330; iron 2.1; copper 0.70; zinc 3.0; chloride 500.

peanuts, excellent source of potassium, calcium, magnesium, phosphorus and sulphur; also the trace minerals iron, copper and zinc. Fresh nuts are low in sodium, but roasting and salting them increases sodium content significantly. Figures given are for fresh and roasted and salted respectively (in mg per 100g): sodium 6, 440; chloride 7, 660. Identical quantities for the following: potassium 680; calcium 61; magnesium 180; phosphorus 370; iron 2.0; copper 0.27; zinc 3.0; sulphur 380.

pears, virtually free of sodium with useful potassium levels. Small amounts of all the other minerals.

Eating variety — raw, edible portion contains levels of the following (in mg per 100g): sodium 2; potassium 130; calcium 8; magnesium 7; phosphorus 10; iron 0.2; copper 0.15; zinc 0.1; sulphur 5; chloride only trace.

Cooking variety, stewed without sugar and with sugar respectively (in mg per 100g): sodium 3, 2; potassium 85, 78; calcium 6, 5; magnesium 3, 3; phosphorus 13, 12; iron 0.2, 0.2; copper 0.09, 0.09; zinc 0.1, 0.1; sulphur 3, 2; chloride 2, 2.

Canned, provides (in mg per 100g): sodium 1; potassium 90; calcium 5; magnesium 6; phosphorus 5; iron 0.3; copper 0.04; sulphur 1; chloride 3.

peas, as grown are virtually free of sodium and a good source of potassium but also supply useful quantities of iron, copper, zinc and phosphorus. Canned peas are high in sodium because of salt addition.

As fresh, raw and boiled respectively (in mg per 100g) contain the following mineral levels: sodium 1, trace; potassium 340, 170; calcium 15, 13; magnesium 30, 21; phosphorus 100, 83; iron 1.9, 1.2; copper 0.23; 0.15; zinc 0.7, 0.5; sulphur 50, 44; chloride 38, 8.

Frozen variety supply (in mg per 100g), raw and boiled respectively: sodium 3, 2; potassium 190, 130; calcium 33, 31; magnesium 27, 23; phosphorus 90, 84; iron 1.5, 1.4; copper 0.22, 0.19; zinc 0.9, 0.7; chloride 20, 12.

Canned peas, as garden and processed respectively supply (in mg per 100g): sodium 230, 330; potassium 130, 170; calcium 24, 27; magnesium 17, 24; phosphorus 73, 91; iron 1.6, 1.5; copper 0.16, 0.22; zinc 0.7, 0.8; chloride 350, 510.

Dried variety supply (in mg per 100g), raw and boiled respectively: sodium 38, 13; potassium 990, 270; calcium 61, 24; magnesium 116, 30; phosphorus 300, 110; iron 4.7, 1.4; copper 0.49, 0.17; zinc 3.5, 1.0; sulphur 130, 39; chloride 60, 9.

---

penta potassium triphosphate, also known as potassium tripolyphosphate. A food additive used as an emulsifying salt, as a texturizer; E450b. Acceptable daily intake up to 350mg per kg body weight. Provides 43.6mg potassium and 20.2mg phosphorus per 100mg. Permitted in some cheeses, in unsweetened condensed-milk products; as a miscellaneous additive.

---

pentasodium triphosphate, a food additive that is an emulsifying salt; a texturizer; E450b. Acceptable daily intake up to 300mg per kg body weight. Provides 31.3mg sodium and 25.3mg phosphorus per 100mg. Permitted in some cheeses; in unsweetened condensed-milk products; in boiler feed water for direct steam treatment of milk; as a miscellaneous additive.

---

peppers, main asset is as good supplier of potassium with virtually no sodium but has small amounts of all other minerals present. Green variety, in raw and boiled state respectively, contain (in mg per 100g): sodium 2, 2; potassium 210, 170; calcium 9, 9; magnesium 11, 10; phosphorus 25, 22; iron 0.4, 0.4; copper 0.07, 0.06; zinc 0.2, 0.2; chloride 18, 15.

---

phosphorus, Chemical symbol P. Atomic weight 30.9. Does not occur free in nature but is found in the form of phosphates (i.e. combined with oxygen) in the minerals chlorapatite, fluorapatite, vivianite, wavellite and phosphate rock or phosphorite. Abundance in the earth's crust is about 0.12 per cent. As phosphate, it is a major constituent of all plant and animal cells and is present in all natural foods. Phosphate is added to many processed foods. Phosphorus intake is between 1.5 and 2.0 grammes per day from a wide variety of food, so dietary deficiency is highly unlikely. A greater possibility is excessive intakes of phosphate from soft drinks, junk foods and processed foods. Animals grazing on lands that are low in phosphate may develop deficiency.

Richest sources of phosphorus in natural foods are (in mg per 100g): yeast extract 1900; dried brewer's yeast 1753; dried skimmed milk 950; wheatgerm 930; soya flour 600; Cheddar cheese 520; canned sardines 520; processed cheese 490; compressed baker's yeast 390; roasted peanuts 370; brown rice 292; evaporated milk 250; wholemeal bread 240; eggs 218; chicken 200; cod 170; beef 150; natural yogurt 140; cottage cheese 140; goat's milk 110; cream cheese 100; white rice 100. All high-protein foods are rich in phosphorus.

Body content of phosphorus parallels that of calcium — a person weighing 70kg (11 stone) contains between 550 and 770g (1.2 and 1.7 lb) phosphorus. Ninety per cent of this is in the bones and teeth as calcium phosphate. Bone is composed of deposits of calcium phosphates within a soft, fibrous organic matrix. The major inorganic component resembles the natural mineral hydroxyapatite. In early life calcium phosphate is of a non-crystalline or amorphous nature but as the child grows the harder, crystalline type predominates. This type is also present in tooth enamel and dentin but crystals are larger, producing greater hardness. Muscle contains 10 per cent of body phosphorus with 1 per cent present in nerve tissue.

Absorption of phosphate from the food depends upon vitamin D which also controls calcium and, to some extent, magnesium absorption. The vitamin is also needed for absorption of phosphate, calcium and magnesium into the bone.

Blood levels of phosphorus are maintained at between 2.5 and 4.5mg per 100ml, mainly by excretion of excess through the kidneys. Decreased blood levels are seen in rickets due to non-absorption of phosphate and in vitamin D-resistant rickets due to defective retention of phosphate by the kidneys.

Dietary relationship between phosphorus and calcium is no longer considered important in their absorption. Once it was believed that the phosphate content of the diet had a crucial influence on calcium absorption because it was known that a high dietary calcium:phosphorus ratio caused rickets in rats. Subsequent human experiments indicated that in breast-fed babies a supplement of phosphates did not interfere with calcium absorption; in adults extra phosphate at a level of between 250 and 1000mg daily for several weeks did not affect calcium balance. Only in babies fed artificial milks in the first few weeks of life can the calcium:phosphorus ratio be important. In human breast milk the ratio is 2:1; in cow's milk it is 1.2:1. The higher level of phosphorus in cow's milk is believed to cause muscular spasm (tetany) in the first week of life in babies fed this food undiluted. Raising the ratio to at least 1.5:1 is considered desirable and this is now carried out on dried milks for babies. In addition, calcium and phosphorus levels of liquid cow's milk are much higher than those of human breast milk so cow's milk levels are adjusted to make them more comparable to those of humans.

Functions of phosphorus are:

1. as phosphates in the structural make-up of bones and teeth;
2. as soluble phosphates in many and varied reactions in the body;
3. as one of the main negatively-charged groups (chloride is the other) that neutralize the positively-charged minerals such as sodium, potassium, calcium and magnesium in body tissues;
4. in the production of energy in all body cells utilizing creative phosphate, adenosine triphosphate and other complexes of phosphates. Removal of high-energy phosphate bands from these substances creates energy for all body processes.
5. to combine with glycogen (animal starch) before its breakdown to glucose and the subsequent burning of glucose to carbon dioxide, water and energy;
6. as cofactor for many enzymes in metabolic body processes;
7. to combine with vitamins of the B complex to produce phosphate complexes that are the active forms of these vitamins;
8. as an essential component of proteins, fats such as lecithin, where it combines with choline and inositol, and of carbohydrates;
9. to combine with dietary constituents to enhance their absorption from the intestine;
10. as monosodium phosphate and disodium phosphate, which are acid and alkaline respectively, in the maintenance of the pH of the blood at the slightly alkaline value of between 7.39 and 7.41;
11. as a constituent of nucleic acids, both ribonucleic (RNA) and deoxyribonucleic (DNA), which are concerned with control of protein synthesis, cell repair and are the basis of heredity and the carriers of genetic information for all living creatures.

Deficiency of phosphorus was once considered highly unlikely for those on modern Western diets, but recent studies of blood phosphate levels in general-hospital patients revealed that more than 2 per cent of them had hypophosphataemia, i.e. low blood phosphate concentration. Profound hypophosphataemia may arise during the first three days of treatment for diabetic ketoacidosis; within one to four days of withdrawal of alcohol in severe alcoholics; from the fourth day onwards in patients receiving intravenous nutrition without phosphate supplements; during the recovery phase after severe burns; during protein and calorie malnutrition; after kidney dialysis if phosphate is not included in the dialysing fluid; during severe respiratory alkalosis; in those taking phosphate binders in excess, such as aluminium hydroxide antacids; in the disease called hypophosphataemic rickets (vitamin D-resistant rickets) characterized by impaired re-absorption of phosphate in the kidneys.

Deficiency symptoms include:

1. debility;
2. loss of appetite;
3. weakness;
4. bone pain;
5. joint stiffness;
6. general malaise;
7. central nervous system disorders such as irritability; muscle weakness; numbness; tingling sensations (paraesthesiae or 'pins and needles'); speech disorders (dysarthria); tremor; confusion; seizures and coma;
8. respiratory failure;
9. heart-muscle weakness (cardiomyopathy);
10. osteomalacia.

All respond to phosphate replacement therapy.

Deficiency effects and consequences include abnormalities of red blood-cell function with depletion of adenosine triphosphate (energy provider) and impaired oxygen transport; haemolysis (splitting of red blood cells) resulting in anaemia; subnormal white blood-cell functions resulting in reduced resistance to infection; depressed platelet (tiny white blood cells) numbers and functions that can upset clotting characteristics of the blood.

Therapy of deficiency is intravenous administration of soluble phosphate (e.g. potassium) in severe cases but blood plasma phosphate, calcium and potassium must be monitored continuously. Oral replacement is usually with one of the supplements mentioned below.

Supplementary forms of phosphorus include bonemeal; sodium phosphate; effervescent phosphate preparations; potassium phosphate; calcium phosphates; calcium glycerophosphate; magnesium glycerophosphate; sodium glycerophosphate.

Recommended dietary intakes of phosphorus have been suggested by the US authorities and are (in mg per day): infants 0-0.5 year, 240; 0.5-1.0

year, 400; children 1-3 yrs, 800; 4-6 yrs, 800; 7-10 yrs, 800; males 11-14 yrs, 1200, 15-18 yrs, 1200; 19-22 yrs, 800; 23-50 yrs, 800; 51 yrs plus, 800; females 11-14 yrs, 1200; 15-18 yrs, 1200; 19-22 yrs, 800; 23-50 yrs, 800; 51 yrs plus, 800; during pregnancy, 1200; whilst breast-feeding, 1200. UK and WHO authorities make no recommendations. For intravenous nutrition the daily allowance is 4.7mg phosphorus per kg body weight.

Excessive oral intakes of phosphorus can prevent the absorption of iron, calcium, magnesium and zinc by formation of insoluble phosphates. Phytic acid, which is inositol hexaphosphoric acid, prevents absorption of these minerals in a similar manner. Too much oral phosphates can cause diarrhoea. If blood levels of phosphate are too high calcification in the soft tissues can occur and blood levels of calcium will fall.

---

phytic acid, also known as inositol hexaphosphate. Provides 28.2mg phosphorus per 100mg. Has long been known to be a constituent of cereals, vegetables and most plant materials. It can combine with metals of nutritional importance to form phytates that are stable in the normal digestive system and so cannot be absorbed. Those most affected are calcium, iron and zinc. There is some evidence that animals, including man, who have high phytic acid intakes can induce an enzyme called phytase which hydrolyses the phytic acid-metal complexes liberating the mineral. The phytic acid content of a normal, balanced diet is unlikely to affect the essential minerals to a significant extent. Problems may arise in those eating high-cereal, high-vegetable content diets where these foods are the sole source of minerals. Examples were seen in young children on a poor diet in Ireland in the 1940s. Phytic acid is concentrated in the aleurone layer of the wheat grain and is present in high concentration in high-extraction flours and in the bran. Phytic acid contents are (in mg per 100g): bran 4225; wholemeal flour 805; white flour 200. These Irish children lived on wholemeal flour products with little dairy produce for three years. The reduced absorption of calcium as a result caused high rates in the incidence of rickets. Reducing the extraction rate of flour to 85 per cent, combined with more milk and dairy products in their diets, caused the rate in incidence of rickets to drop. Similar problems have been encountered with Asian immigrants in the UK. Although low vitamin D levels in the body was the main cause of the increased incidence of rickets and osteomalacia, high intakes of phytic acid in chapathis and low intake of calcium from dairy sources were also factors.

In the preparation of bread, much of the phytic acid content of the flour is destroyed. The traditional long-proving technique of breadmaking causes 50 per cent of the phytic acid of wholemeal bread to be destroyed. Techniques that use shorter proving times, like those utilizing vitamin C, give rise to losses of phytic acid totalling one-third of that in the original wholemeal flour. Most destruction is due to the enzyme phytase present in wheat and in yeast. Once this is inactivated by the baking process, further destruction is initiated by the high oven temperature.

Problems with phytic acid are more likely to arise with high intakes of raw bran, cereals and vegetables. The main source is high extraction flours but oats, high-bran breakfast foods, soya and other beans also contribute meaningful quantities of phytic acid. When the phytate:zinc ratio in these diets exceeds 15:1, the availability of zinc decreases drastically. The zinc in wholemeal bread is 3.0mg per 100g but is less readily available than that in white bread which is only 0.9mg per 100g. This is less important in the UK where three-quarters of the zinc in the diet comes from animal, fish and dairy-based foods than in those countries where cereals and vegetables supply the greater part of dietary zinc.

Table 10 indicates the zinc, phytic acid and dietary fibre contents of cereal foods. Ratios of greater than 15 reduce zinc bioavailability.

Table 10: Zinc, phytic acid and dietary fibre contents of cereal foods

Cereal food	Zinc mg/100g	Phytic acid mg/100g	Phytic acid Zinc under ratio	Dietary fibre g/100g
Wholemeal flour	2.4	850	35	9.6
White flour	1.5	200	13	7.5
Wholemeal bread	1.8	610	33	8.5
Brown bread	1.8	440	25	5.1
White bread	0.6	90	15	2.7
Bran-based cereals	3.6	2200	60	26.7
Cornflakes	0.3	60	21	11.0
Wheat-based cereals	2.8	820	29	12.3
Oatmeal	3.4	940	27	7.0

Meat extenders and replacers derived from soya beans can also provide phytic acid which can bind zinc. This is illustrated in Table 11. Ratios of greater than 15 decrease zinc bioavailability.

Table 11: Phytic acid produced from meat extenders and replacers

Product on a dry weight basis	Zinc (mg/100g)	Phytic acid (g/100g)	Molar ratio Phytic acid:zinc
Meat extender	4.3	1.6	37
Mince additive	3.5	1.4	39
TVP beef	4.2	1.3	31
TVP pork	4.1	1.8	43
TVP mince	5.0	1.8	36
TVP unflavoured	4.4	1.9	43
Beef	17.0 (av.)	0	—
Pork	6.6 (av.)	0	—

piccalilli, very rich in sodium as added salt. Small quantities of all other minerals present. It provides the following mineral levels (in mg per 100g): sodium 1200; potassium 55; calcium 24; magnesium 10; phosphorus 23; iron 0.9; copper 0.10; zinc 0.2; chloride 1700.

pineapple, virtually sodium free with good levels of potassium plus small amounts of all other minerals present. Figures for fresh and canned respectively (in mg per 100g): sodium 2, 1; potassium 250, 94; calcium 12, 13; magnesium 17, 8; phosphorus 8, 5; iron 0.4, 0.4; copper 0.08, 0.05; zinc 0.1, 0; sulphur 3, 3; chloride 29, 4.

pineapple juice, main attribute is good supplier of potassium with small but useful amounts of all other minerals. When canned provides the following levels (in mg per 100g): sodium 1; potassium 140; calcium 12; magnesium 12; phosphorus 10; iron 0.7; copper 0.09; chloride 38.

plantain, very rich source of potassium with traces only of sodium present. Useful supplier of all other minerals. Mineral levels for raw, boiled and fried respectively (in mg per 100g): sodium 1, 4, 3; potassium 350, 330, 610; calcium 7, 9, 6; magnesium 33, 34, 54; phosphorus 35, 34, 66; iron 0.5, 0.4, 0.8; copper 0.16, 0.1, 0.2; zinc 0.1, 0.2, 0.4; sulphur 15 for raw state only; chloride 80, 50, 110.

Plummer's disease, *see* hyperthyroidism.

---

plums, small quantities of most minerals but a good source of potassium with negligible sodium content.

Victoria dessert variety provides quantities of the following for raw, edible portion (in mg per 100g): sodium 2; potassium 190; calcium 11; magnesium 7; phosphorus 16; iron 0.4; copper 0.10; zinc trace; sulphur 4; chloride trace.

Cooking variety supplies levels for stewed without sugar and with sugar respectively (in mg per 100g): sodium 2, 2; potassium 160, 150; calcium 12, 11; magnesium 6, 5; phosphorus 12, 11; iron 0.3, 0.2; copper 0.08, 0.06; zinc, a trace in both states; sulphur, identical in both forms, 3; chloride, trace found in both states.

---

pomegranate juice, good supplier of potassium with traces of all the other minerals. It provides the following quantities (in mg per 100g): sodium 1; potassium 200; calcium 3; magnesium 3; phosphorus 8; iron 0.2; copper 0.07; sulphur 4; chloride 53.

---

pork, good content of iron, copper and zinc but particularly rich in potassium, sulphur and phosphorus. Moderate amount of sodium, augmented by addition of salt. All cuts when cooked supply mineral levels (in mg per 100g) in the range: sodium 79-95; potassium 210-420; calcium 9-11; magnesium 9-29; phosphorus 110-260; iron 1.0-1.3; copper 0.15-0.29; zinc 0.9-3.5; sulphur 300-310; chloride 76-92.

---

port, small quantities of most minerals but supplies useful amounts of potassium and iron. Minerals present are (in mg per 100ml): sodium 4; potassium 97; calcium 4; magnesium 11; phosphorus 12; iron 0.40; copper 0.10; chloride 8.

---

potassium, chemical symbol K, from the Latin *kalium*. Atomic weight 39.1. Alkali metal that is found mainly as sylvite (potassium chloride) and in the aluminosilicates orthoclase and microcline and as carnallite. Occurrence in earth's crust is 2.59 per cent.

The body potassium content of a person weighing 65kg is about 140g. Of this, only 3.1g is present in the extracellular fluid. The remaining 137g occurs inside body cells and of this, four-fifths is present in skeletal muscles. The quantity in the skeleton is negligible.

Dietary intakes of potassium are between 1960 and 5870mg daily with a usual intake of 2.54g equivalent to 4.85g potassium chloride.

Food sources of potassium are widespread but very variable in content. The best sources are (in mg per 100g): dried fruits 710-1880; soya flour 1660-2030; molasses 1470; wheat bran 1160; raw salad vegetables 140-1080; chipped potatoes 1020; nuts 350-940; breakfast cereals and mueslis 100-600; savoury biscuits 140-500; fresh fruit 65-430; boiled vegetables 50-400; fish 230-360; meat and poultry 33-350; fruit juices 110-260; wholemeal flour 360; wholemeal bread 220; white bread 100; eggs 140; cheese 100-190; brown rice 190; polished rice 110. Beverages are particularly rich sources, e.g. instant coffee 4000; Indian tea 2160; roasted coffee 2020; cocoa powder 1500; drinking chocolate 410. For other levels see individual foods.

Absorption of potassium from the diet is passive requiring no specific mechanism. Absorption takes place throughout the small intestine and is dependent on the potassium concentration within the intestinal contents. Absorption takes place as long as this concentration is greater than that of the blood. Secretion of potassium probably takes place in the large bowel. Required movement of intestine contents through the small and large intestine is unfavourable to absorption. Under these conditions, such as persistent diarrhoea, low body potassium can develop.

Excretion of potassium reflects its dietary intake. Out of a daily intake of 2.35g, 2.15g is excreted in the urine with 0.39g in the faeces. The negative balance of 0.19g is due to normal cellular breakdown which releases potassium eventually into the urine. Such breakdown of cellular proteins increases in diabetes, underfeeding and after injury. Potassium can also be displaced from the cells by hydrogen ions. Any condition giving rise to acidosis is thus liable to cause cellular depletion of potassium.

Diuretic drugs, particularly the thiazide variety, act by increasing the output of sodium and water from the kidneys but at the same time potassium excretion is increased. Supplementation with this is therefore usual. In severe kidney failure, potassium is not excreted in the urine and excessive levels build up in the blood and tissue. The consequences are discussed below.

Faecal excretion is low in a healthy person, probably not exceeding 200mg daily. The digestive juices contain significant amounts but these are usually re-absorbed in the lower gut. Diarrhoea can cause large losses in the faeces in amounts of up to 3.52g in 24 hours. This is particularly serious in infants suffering from diarrhoea induced by protein-energy malnutrition who may lose as much as 10-30 per cent of total body potassium. Heart failure may result. Similar losses may appear in infants or adults with chronic diarrhoea brought on by other causes (e.g. infection) and it is important in these cases that potassium as well as water losses are replaced by supplementation.

Sweat losses of potassium are usually negligible since sweat contains only about 352mg per litre. Excessive perspiration can lead to more significant losses but these do not approach those of sodium in importance.

Functions of potassium are:
1.   in maintaining a normal balance of water within body cells as the major positively-charged ion within these cells;
2.   as an essential activator in a number of enzymes particularly those concerned with energy production;
3.   to help stabilize the internal structure of body cells;
4.   in assisting specialized cell particles to synthesize proteins;
5.   in nerve impulse transmission in conjunction with sodium;
6.   to increase the excitability of heart and skeletal muscle to make them more receptive to nerve impulses;
7.   in preserving the acid-alkali balance of the body in conjunction with bicarbonate, phosphate and protein as well as with sodium, calcium and magnesium;
8.   in stimulating the normal movements of the intestinal tract.

Causes of potassium deficiency are:
1.   drug therapy with: (a) thiazide and other diuretics including frusemide, chlorthalidone, ethacrynic acid, mercurials and carbonic anhydrase inhibitors; (b) long-term use of corticosteroids and ACTH; (c) overuse of laxatives; (d) excessive intake of liquorice and the drug carbenoxolene from liquorice; (e) high-dose sodium penicillin and carbenicillin; (f) intravenous infusions of glucose and salt solutions not containing potassium; (g) ion-exchange resins used to reduce blood cholesterol; (h) low sodium diets.
2.   surgical operations — ileostomy, colostomy; extensive bowel resection; gastric drainage. Other deficiency causes are extensive burns; extensive injury; diabetes mellitus; Cushing's syndrome; excessive excretion of aldosterone; diabetes insipidus; periodic familial paralysis; chronic diarrhoea; persistent vomiting; influenza; megaloblastic anaemia; ulcerative colitis; kidney disease; severe heart disease; chronic respiratory failure; prolonged fasting; therapeutic starvation; bizarre diets, especially in the elderly; anorexia nervosa; alcoholism; clay eating; cystic fibrosis; alkalosis.

Symptoms of deficiency include vomiting; abdominal distension; paralytic ileus; acute muscular weakness; paralysis; paraesthesia ('pins and needles'); loss of appetite; low blood pressure; polydipsia (intense thirst); drowsiness and confusion leading to respiratory failure; coma; an inability to concentrate urine; increased toxicity of digitalis.

Treatment of low potassium levels is with:

1. oral or intravenous potassium chloride solutions;
2. increased dietary intake of potassium-rich foods;
3. drugs such as triamterene or spironolactone taken with potassium-losing diuretics.

Potassium phosphate may be given by injection as an alternative to potassium chloride in the presence of acidosis.

Excess of potassium causes effects first on the muscles of the skeleton and of the heart, giving rise to muscular weakness and mental apathy. Intravenous potassium in excess may stop the heart. High oral doses can cause ulceration of the small bowel, particularly if the tablets are of the enteric-coated type (i.e. treated to prevent dissolution in the stomach to ensure they dissolve in the small intestine) which produce a localized high concentration of potassium. Lower doses of salts may cause nausea, vomiting, diarrhoea and abdominal cramps.

Causes of potassium excess include kidney failure; insufficient production of adrenal gland hormones; shock after injury in which condition potassium leaks out of the damaged cells into the blood. Treatment is withdrawal of potassium salts and of foods; in serious cases medical expertise is necessary.

Supplementary form of potassium is usually potassium chloride which provides 52.4mg potassium in 100mg chloride but potassium acetate, bicarbonate, citrate, gluconate, sulphate, acid tartrate, tartrate and phosphates have also been used (see individual salts). Amino acid or protein complexes are also available which are claimed to be better absorbed than potassium salts. These complexes also replace protein losses which may accompany excessive potassium excretion.

Food additives that contain potassium are: potassium acetate; potassium alginate; potassium benzoate; potassium bromate; potassium carbonate; potassium chloride; tripotassium citrate; tetrapotassium diphosphate; potassium ferrocyanide; potassium gluconate; potassium bicarbonate; potassium dihydrogen citrate; potassium hydrogen glutamate; potassium dihydrogen orthophosphate; dipotassium hydrogen orthophosphate; potassium hydroxide; potassium lactate; potassium malate; potassium metabisulphite; potassium nitrate; potassium nitrite; tripotassium orthophosphate; potassium pectate; potassium persulphate; potassium polyphosphates; potassium propionate; potassium salts of fatty acids; potassium sodium tartrate; potassium sorbate; potassium sulphate; dipotassium tartrate; monopotassium tartrate; pentapotassium triphosphate.

---

potassium acetate,   provides 40mg potassium in 100mg acetate. Used as oral and injectable supplement and in solutions for kidney dialysis. It increases alkali reserve making the urine less acid. Has been used as a diuretic. Has a mild diaphoretic action (induces sweating). Usual dose is 1-2g as required.

Also used as a food additive, E261. Functions as a buffer; as a preservative. Acceptable daily intake is not limited. Permitted as a miscellaneous additive.

---

potassium acid phosphate,   also known as monobasic potassium phosphate; potassium biphosphate; potassium dihydrogen orthophosphate. Provides 28.7mg potassium and 22.8mg phosphorus in 100mg phosphate. Used as a mild purgative in dilute solution as it causes retention of water in the bowel giving rise to evacuation within 1-2 hrs. Used also in the treatment of calcium and phosphate metabolic disorders. Usual dose is 1-4g as required.

---

potassium acid tartrate,   also known as cream of tartar; potassium hydrogen tartrate. Provides 20.8mg potassium in 100mg acid tartrate. Used as a saline purgative. Has a mild diuretic action. Usual dose is 1-4g as required. Also accepted as a food additive.

---

potassium alginate,   a food additive, E402, that functions as an emulsifier or stabilizer; as a gelling agent; as a boiler water additive. Acceptable daily intake up to 50mg per kg body weight. Permitted as diluent for food colours; in boiler feed water for direct steam treatment of milk; as stabilizer or emulsifier; in reduced-sugar jam products.

---

potassium benzoate,   a food additive that is used as a preservative,

E214. Provides 18.3mg potassium per 100mg. Acceptable daily intake up to 5mg per kg body weight. Permitted as a preservative in certain foods, quantity restricted.

potassium bicarbonate, provides 39.0mg potassium in 100mg bicarbonate. Used as potassium supplement in mixtures and in effervescent tablets. Has been used as an antacid; as a diuretic; to make the urine less acid. Usual dose is 1-2g as required. Also allowed as a food additive. Acceptable daily intake is not limited. Permitted in certain cocoa products; in condensed-milk and dried-milk products; in certain wines; as a miscellaneous additive.

potassium bromate, a food additive used only as an improving agent for flour. Acceptable daily intake up to 20mg per kg; from 20-75mg per kg for special purposes. Provides 23.4mg potassium and 47.9mg bromine per 100mg. Permitted in bread and flour other than wholemeal.

potassium carbonate, a food additive used as an alkali. Acceptable daily intake is not limited. Provides 56.7mg per 100mg. Permitted in sterilized and UHT cream; in certain cocoa products; in boiler feed water for direct steam treatment of milk; as a miscellaneous additive.

potassium chloride, a food additive. Functions as a gelling agent; a salt substitute; dietary supplement for potassium and chloride. Acceptable daily intake is not limited. Provides 52.5mg potassium and 47.7mg chloride per 100mg. Permitted as a miscellaneous additive.

potassium dihydrogen citrate, a food additive, E332, used as a buffer; as an emulsifying salt. Acceptable daily intake is not limited. Provides 17.0mg potassium per 100mg. Permitted in sterilized and UHT cream; in some cheeses; in condensed milk and dried-milk products; in reduced-sugar jam products; as a miscellaneous additive.

potassium dihydrogen orthophosphate, also known as monobasic potassium phosphate. Used as a food additive as a sequestrant; as a buffer; as an emulsifying salt; E340. Acceptable daily intake 307mg per kg body weight at normal calcium intake. Provides 28.8mg potassium and 22.8mg phosphorus per 100mg. Permitted in sterilized and UHT cream; in some cheeses; in condensed-milk and dried-milk products; as a miscellaneous additive.

potassium ferrocyanide, also known as potassium hexacyanoferrate II. Used as a food additive to prevent caking of powders, e.g. salt. Acceptable daily intake up to 0.025mg per kg body weight. Provides 37.1mg potassium and 13.3mg iron per 100mg. Permitted in certain wines; as a miscellaneous additive.

potassium gluconate, provides 16.7mg potassium in 100mg gluconate. Used as oral supplement with the advantage of being almost tasteless. Claimed to be better absorbed than other potassium salts. Usual dose is from 5-10g daily. Acceptable daily intake is up to 50mg per kg body weight. Also allowed as a food additive.

potassium glycerophosphate, liquid preparation providing 12.5mg phosphorus and 31.5mg potassium per 100mg glycerophosphate. Dose is usually 0.6-2.0g up to a daily intake of 6g. Used mainly as a tonic.

potassium hydrogen L-glutamate, a food additive used as a flavour enhancer; as a salt substitute. Acceptable daily intake is up to 120mg per kg body weight; not to be given to infants under 12 weeks old. Provides 20.9mg potassium per 100mg. Permitted only in dietetic foods.

potassium hydroxide, a food additive used as an alkali. Acceptable daily intake is not limited. Provides 69.8mg potassium per 100mg. Permitted in certain cocoa products; as a miscellaneous additive.

potassium iodate, provides 59.3µg iodine in 100µg iodate. Has been used as additive to dough in breadmaking at a level of 2mg per kilogram bread to prevent endemic goitre. The daily iodide intake was between 80 and 270µg. Has also been used to iodize table salt at a level of 1mg per 40g salt (about 1½ ounces) to prevent goitre. It is not a permitted additive to dough in the UK.

potassium iodide, provides 76.5µg iodine in 100µg iodide. Used as a supplement in areas of endemic goitre. Supplementary daily dose is 200µg to 1200µg potassium iodide.

In larger doses (150mg daily) it is given in pre-operative treatment of thyrotoxicosis. At 250-500mg dose it is an expectorant. It should not be given in pulmonary tuberculosis as it may convert a dormant into an active disease.

Toxic effects of excess potassium iodide and iodides in general are mental depression; nervousness; insomnia; sexual impotence; myxoedema; goitre in adults and in infants born to mothers taking iodides.

potassium lactate, a food additive used as a buffer; as an antioxidant; as a synergist. Acceptable daily intake is not limited. Provides 30.5mg potassium per 100mg. Permitted in reduced-sugar jam products; as a miscellaneous additive.

potassium malate, a food additive used as a buffer. Acceptable daily intake is not limited. Provides 37.2mg potassium per 100mg. Permitted in reduced-sugar jam products; as a miscellaneous additive.

potassium metabisulphite, also known as potassium disulphite; potassium pyrophosphate. A food additive used as a preservative, E224. Acceptable daily intake is up to 0.7mg per kg body weight. Provides 35.2mg potassium and 14.4mg sulphur per 100mg. Permitted in most specified sugar products; in certain fruit juices; in certain wines.

potassium metaphosphate, also known as potassium polymetaphosphate; potassium Kurrol's salt. Used as a buffering agent; as a fat emulsifier; as a moisture-retaining agent in processed foods.

potassium molybdate, provides 40.3µg molybdenum and 32.8µg potassium in 100µg molybdate. Daily intake of potassium molybdate should not exceed 0.5mg when used as a supplement as the substance is toxic in large quantities.

potassium nitrate, also known as saltpetre. A food additive used as a preservative; as a curing salt; E252. Acceptable daily intake up to 5mg per kg body weight. Provides 38.7mg potassium in 100mg. Permitted in cured meats; in some cheeses. May not be added to foods made for young children and babies.

potassium nitrite, a food additive used as a preservative; as a curing agent; E249. Acceptable daily intake up to 0.2mg per kg body weight. Provides 46.0mg potassium per 100mg. Permitted in cured meats; in some cheeses. May not be added to food for babies and young children.

potassium orthophosphate, also known as tribasic potassium phosphate. A food additive used as a buffer; as an emulsifying salt; E340. Acceptable daily intake up to 300mg per kg body weight. Provides 55.3mg potassium and 29.2mg phosphorus per 100mg. Permitted in sterilized and UHT cream; in some cheeses; in condensed-milk and dried-milk products; as a miscellaneous additive.

potassium pectate, a food additive used as an emulsifier or stabilizer; as a gelling agent; E440a. Acceptable daily intake is not specified. Permitted as an emulsifier or stabilizer; in certain jam products.

potassium persulphate, a food additive used as a flour-improving agent. Acceptable daily intake has not been set. Provides 29.0mg potassium and 23.7mg sulphur per 100mg. Permitted in flour or bread other than wholemeal.

potassium phosphate, also known as dibasic potassium phosphate; dipotassium monophosphate; dipotassium phosphate; dipotassium hydrogen orthophosphate. Provides 33.3mg potassium and 17.8mg phosphorus in 100mg phosphate. Usual dose is 0.6-2.0g as required. For uses *see* potassium acid phosphate.

---

potassium polyphosphates,   food additives used as emulsifying salts; as stabilizers; E450c. Acceptable daily intake up to 350mg per kg body weight. Permitted in some cheeses; in unsweetened condensed-milk products; as a miscellaneous additive.

---

potassium propionate,   a food additive used as a preservative, E283. Acceptable daily limit is not limited. Provides 34.9mg potassium per 100mg. Permitted in bread; in flour confectionery; in Christmas pudding, quantity restricted.

---

potassium soaps,   also known as potassium salts of fatty acids. Food additives used as emulsifiers; stabilizers; E470. Acceptable daily intakes not limited. Permitted to contain certain antioxidants; as emulsifiers and stabilizers; in Dutch rusks.

---

potassium sodium tartrate,   a food additive also known as Rochelle salt. Functions as a buffer; as an emulsifying salt; E282. Provides 13.9mg potassium and 8.2mg sodium per 100mg. Permitted in some cheeses; as a miscellaneous additive. Acceptable daily intake up to 30mg per kg body weight.

---

potassium sorbate,   a food additive used as a preservative, E202. Acceptable daily intake up to 0.25mg per kg body weight. Provides 26.1mg potassium per 100mg. Permitted in certain foods; in certain wines, quantity restricted.

---

potassium sulphate,   provides 44.9mg potassium and 18.4mg sulphur in 100mg. Used as a saline purgative in dilute solution. Strong solutions are irritating to the stomach and intestines. Usual dose is 1-3g as required. Also accepted as a food additive.

---

potatoes, as they are an important item in the Western diet because of the amount eaten, potatoes in all forms are regarded as supplying significant quantities of potassium, phosphorus, sulphur and chloride plus the trace minerals iron, copper and zinc.

Raw potatoes when old contain the following levels of minerals (in mg per 100g): sodium 7; potassium 570; calcium 8; magnesium 24; phosphorus 40; iron 0.5; copper 0.15; zinc 0.3; sulphur 35; chloride 79.

Boiled, old potatoes contain (in mg per 100g): sodium 3; potassium 330; calcium 4; magnesium 15; phosphorus 29; iron 0.3; copper 0.11; zinc 0.2; sulphur 22; chloride 41.

In the mashed state they contain (in mg per 100g): sodium 24; potassium 300; calcium 12; magnesium 14; phosphorus 32; iron 0.3; copper 0.10; zinc 0.3; sulphur 24; chloride 71.

Baked potatoes contain the following levels, with and without skins (in mg per 100g) respectively: sodium 8, 6; potassium 680, 550; calcium 9, 8; phosphorus 48, 39; iron 0.8, 0.6; copper 0.18, 0.15; zinc 0.3, 0.2; sulphur 42, 34; chloride 94, 76.

As *roast* (in mg per 100g): sodium 9; potassium 750; calcium 10; magnesium 32; phosphorus 53; iron 0.7; copper 0.20; zinc 0.4; sulphur 56; chloride 100.

Chips (in mg per 100g) contain the following: sodium 12; potassium 1020; calcium 14; magnesium 43; phosphorus 72; iron 0.9; copper 0.27; zinc 0.6; sulphur 45; chloride 140.

Crisps have higher levels of the following minerals (in mg per 100g): sodium 550; potassium 1190; calcium 37; magnesium 56; phosphorus 130; iron 2.1; copper 0.22; zinc 0.8; chloride 890.

As *dried* and *made-up mash* respectively (in mg per 100g): sodium 1190, 260; potassium 1550, 340; calcium 89, 20; magnesium 69, 15; phosphorus 220, 48; iron 2.4, 0.5; copper 0.37, 0.08; zinc 1.1, 0.2; chloride 1750, 380.

New, boiled and canned respectively (in mg per 100g): sodium 41, 260; potassium 330, 230; calcium 5, 11; magnesium 20, 10; phosphorus 33, 31; iron 0.4, 0.7; copper 0.15, 0.08; zinc 0.3, 0.3; sulphur 24, 0; chloride 46, 440.

---

prostate gland, the male accessory gland that rests just below the bladder and completely surrounds the bladder's narrow neck called the urethra. When it is enlarged, the prostate pinches off the urethra, restricting the flow of urine. When the prostate is inflamed prostatitis is the result, requiring anti-bacterial treatment. Enlarged prostate, from whatever reason, is usually treated by surgery. Maintaining a healthy prostate appears to require adequate zinc intakes. Both the healthy prostate and the semen usually contain high concentrations of zinc. Those with prostate problems almost invariably had low zinc levels in the gland and in their semen. Supplementation with an average of 25mg elemental zinc daily relieved the symptoms in some men with enlarged prostates. More importantly, adequate intakes of the mineral throughout life may cut down the chances of developing an enlarged prostate. Low saturated-fat diets combined with high-fibre intakes may also contribute.

---

prunes,   excellent source of potassium and iron with significant amounts of calcium, magnesium and phosphorus. Very low in sodium. Mineral quantities for raw, edible portion, stewed without sugar and with sugar respectively (in mg per 100g) are: sodium 12, 7, 5; potassium 860, 440, 420; calcium 38, 19, 18; magnesium 38, 13, 13; phosphorus 83, 42, 40; iron 2.9, 1.4, 1.4; copper 0.16, 0.08, 0.08; sulphur 19, 9, 9; chloride 3, 1, 1.

---

psoriatic arthritis,   a particular form of arthritis that is associated with the skin complaint psoriasis. Occurs in a minority of those with psoriasis but is very painful and disabling. May occur in spine, toes and fingers as a spondylitis; in back joints as sacroiliitis. Studies in Denmark indicate that some cases respond to the mineral zinc, taken as zinc sulphate (220mg, three times daily). Stiff joints became mobile; grip strengthened; swelling was reduced; pain and morning stiffness disappeared. Benefit may be due to the activity of zinc in the body's own immune system that attacks the inflammatory response in arthritis. The skin complaint psoriasis may also respond.

---

pudding,   when made with milk is an excellent provider of calcium, phosphorus and potassium; low in sodium. Yorkshire variety provides good amounts of potassium, calcium, phosphorus and iron but is also high in sodium because of added salt.

Milk variety supplies the following minerals (in mg per 100g): sodium 55; potassium 160; calcium 130; magnesium 14; phosphorus 110; iron 0.1; copper 0.03; sulphur 37; chloride 110.

Canned rice variety provides levels (in mg per 100g) of: sodium 50, potassium 140; calcium 93; magnesium 11; phosphorus 80; iron 0.2; copper 0.03; zinc 0.4; chloride 95.

Yorkshire supplies (in mg per 100g): sodium 600; potassium 160; calcium 130; magnesium 20; phosphorus 130; iron 1.0; copper 0.08; zinc 0.7; chloride 94.

pumpkin, useful calcium and trace minerals content, but rich source of potassium, and sodium free. In raw state it provides the following mineral levels (in mg per 100g): sodium 1; potassium 310; calcium 39; magnesium 8, phosphorus 19; iron 0.4; copper 0.08; zinc 0.2; sulphur 10; chloride 37.

Q

quinces, small amounts of most minerals but they contain good quantity of potassium. As raw they supply (in mg per 100g): sodium 3; potassium 200; calcium 14; magnesium 6; phosphorus 19; iron 0.3; copper 0.13; sulphur 5; chloride 2.

R

radishes, good source of iron and potassium. They provide moderate intakes of calcium, sodium, phosphorus and sulphur. Levels of the following minerals (in mg per 100g) are: sodium 59; potassium 240; calcium 44; magnesium 11; phosphorus 27; iron 1.9; copper 0.13; zinc 0.1; sulphur 38; chlorine 19.

raisins, very rich in potassium and a good source of iron, copper, calcium, magnesium and phosphorus. Moderate sodium source. They provide the following minerals (in mg per 100g): sodium 52; potassium 860; calcium 61; magnesium 42; phosphorus 33; iron 1.6; copper 0.24; zinc 0.1; sulphur 23; chloride 9.

raspberries, very low sodium food that is a good source of potassium iron and copper. Useful supplies of calcium, magnesium and phosphorus. As raw, stewed without sugar, stewed with sugar and canned respectively, they contain (in mg per 100g): sodium 3, 3, 3, 4; potassium 220, 230, 210, 100; calcium 41, 43, 39, 14; magnesium 22, 23, 21, 11; phosphorus 29, 31, 28, 14; iron 1.2, 1.3, 1.1, 1.7; copper 0.21, 0.22, 0.20, 0.10; sulphur 17, 18, 16 (no information available for sulphur content in canned state); chloride 22, 23, 21, 5.

recommended dietary intakes, *see* Table 12.

red cabbage, provides significant levels of calcium and sulphur. Rich source of potassium with low sodium content. In raw state it provides the following minerals (in mg per 100g): sodium 32; potassium 300; calcium 53; magnesium 17; phosphorus 32; iron 0.6; copper 0.09; zinc 0.3; sulphur 68; chloride 45.

redcurrants, good source of potassium and iron with moderate quantities of calcium, phosphorus and sulphur. Mineral levels are given for raw, stewed without sugar and stewed with sugar respectively (in mg per 100g): sodium, identical in all states, 2; potassium 280, 240, 220; calcium 36, 31, 28; magnesium 13, 11, 10; phosphorus 30, 26, 23; iron 1.2, 1.0, 0.9; copper 0.12, 0.10, 0.09; zinc 0.12, 0.10, 0.09; sulphur 29, 25, 23; chloride 14, 12, 11.

red kidney beans, excellent supplier of all minerals, including iron, copper and zinc. Particularly rich in potassium with low sodium content. As raw they supply levels (in mg per 100g) of: sodium 40; potassium 1160; calcium 140; magnesium 180; phosphorus 410; iron 6.7; copper 0.61; zinc 2.8; sulphur 170; chloride 2.

Table 12: Recommended dietary intakes of minerals for adults

	Au	Ca	Cz	Dn	FDR	Fi	GDR	H	I	Ne	No	NZ	Po	Ro	Sp	Sw	UK	USA	USSR	WHO/FAO
CALCIUM Female / (mg) Male	700-800	700-800	800	800	700-800	600-700	800	500	600	800	800	800	800	900	400-500	800	500	800	800	600-700
IODINE Female / (µg) Male	150	100-150	—	—	—	—	—	—	—	—	—	150	—	—	—	—	—	150	—	—
IRON Female / (mg) Male	15-12	10-14	14-12	18-10	18-12	12-18	15-10 / 18-12	18-12	18-10	12-10	18-10	15-12	12-12	20-12	14-28	18-10	12-10	18-10	15	14-28
MAGNESIUM Female / (mg) Male	—	250-300 / 350-400	—	300-350	220-260	—	—	—	300-350	—	—	—	300-400	—	—	—	—	300-350	400-600	—
ZINC Female / (mg) Male	—	9-12	8	15	—	—	—	—	15	—	—	—	—	—	—	—	—	15	—	—

Key:

Au:	Australia
Ca:	Canada
Cz:	Czechoslovakia
Dn:	Denmark
FDR:	West Germany
Fi:	Finland
GDR:	East Germany
H:	Hungary
I:	Italy
Ne:	Netherlands
No:	Norway
NZ:	New Zealand
Po:	Poland
Ro:	Romania
Sp:	Spain
Sw:	Sweden
UK:	United Kingdom
USA:	United States of America
USSR:	Russia
FAO:	Food and Agricultural Organization
WHO:	World Health Organization

rhubarb,   rich in potassium and calcium with significant quantities of all other minerals. Mineral levels are given for raw, stewed without sugar, stewed with sugar respectively (in mg per 100g): sodium, identical in all states, 2; potassium 430, 400, 350; calcium 100, 93, 84; magnesium 14, 13, 12; phosphorus 21, 19, 18; iron 0.4, 0.4, 0.3; copper 0.13, 0.12, 0.11; sulphur 8, 7, 7; chloride 87, 81, 73.

---

roe,   rich source of potassium, phosphorus and sulphur with significant levels of iron and chloride. Moderate amount of sodium present.

For *hard* variety, fried, mineral levels are (in mg per 100g): sodium 130; potassium 260; calcium 17; magnesium 11; phosphorus 500; iron 1.6; sulphur 240; chloride 190.

For *soft* variety, fried (in mg per 100g): sodium 87; potassium 240; calcium 16; magnesium 8; phosphorus 920; iron 1.5; sulphur 240; chloride 120.

---

runner beans,   main mineral supplied is potassium; small but significant quantities of calcium, magnesium, phosphorus and the trace elements. When boiled they supply (in mg per 100g): sodium 1; potassium 150; calcium 22; magnesium 17; phosphorus 41; iron 0.7; copper 0.05; zinc 0.3; chloride 5.

---

rye flour,   excellent source of trace minerals with significant quantities of potassium, phosphorus, magnesium and calcium. Contains the following levels of minerals (in mg per 100g): sodium 1; potassium 410; calcium 32; magnesium 92; phosphorus 360; iron 2.7; copper 0.42; zinc 2.8.

S

---

sago,   in the raw state is a good source of iron but little else. It provides (in mg per 100g): sodium 3; potassium 5; calcium 10; magnesium 3;

phosphorus 29; iron 1.2; copper 0.03; sulphur 1; chloride 13. For contents in pudding *see* pudding.

---

salsify, species of goat's-beard cultivated for its root which tastes of asparagus. Good source of potassium, calcium, phosphorus, sulphur, and of trace elements iron and copper. In boiled state, it provides the following minerals (in mg per 100g): sodium 8; potassium 180; calcium 60; magnesium 14; phosphorus 53; iron 1.2; copper 0.12; sulphur 25; chloride 46.

---

salt, strictly speaking a salt is a combination of a metallic element or ammonia with an acid group. Examples are sodium sulphate, potassium chloride, magnesium acetate, calcium phosphate, ammonium chloride, potassium iodide, zinc carbonate, sodium bicarbonate, sodium citrate, potassium tartrate. In these cases, the part of the salt of most interest to the body is the metallic or ammonia bit but chloride, iodide and phosphate can also be utilized because they contain chlorine, iodine and phosphorus respectively.

In common parlance though, salt has come to mean sodium chloride or common salt since this is the most widespread in our diet. When dissolved in water, sodium chloride splits into positively-charged sodium ions (cations) that are electrically neutralized by negatively-charged chloride ions (anions). Hence salt is neutral because there are equal numbers of sodium and chloride ions. All other water-soluble salts split when in solution into positively-charged metal or ammonia ions and negatively-charged acid group ions.

Each 100mg sodium chloride contains 39.3mg sodium and 60.7mg chloride. Salt is the main source of both sodium and chloride in the diet. Other sodium salts present in the diet include sodium bicarbonate, sodium nitrite, monosodium glutamate, sodium benzoate, sodium alginate and sodium sulphite. Like sodium chloride, these too are in the main added to foods. For their sodium contribution to the diet see the individual salt. All foods contain an inherent amount of sodium in them but there are wide variations in the quantity. See the individual foods for their sodium content.

Salt requirements are relatively low. It is doubtful if salt need be added to any food for its nutritional value. There is evidence that early man managed and some primitive communities today manage to survive on a diet to which no salt was or is added. Intakes of natural sodium expressed as sodium chloride are as little as between 30 and 600mg salt per day and these primitive communities have adapted to such small quantities. As civilization progressed man discovered that salt evaporated from sea water or mined from the ground could be used to preserve food. This assumed importance for storing food out of season so salt became highly valued. Roman soldiers were paid partly in salt, hence the word 'salary' for remuneration. As methods for isolating salt improved and as its transport became easier the mineral was cheaper and available to all. Its consumption increased, not because it was needed but because of its flavour-enhancing qualities. Today the population in the West consumes between 8 and 14g salt daily. They could equally well manage on 3.5-7.0g salt daily. High salt consumption leading to high blood levels can be harmful in several conditions (*see under* sodium) but the most important is on blood pressure which is a factor in the development of heart attacks, strokes and kidney failure.

Dietary salt and high blood pressure appear to be related on the basis of animal experiments and epidemiological studies. In animals with inherent forms of high blood pressure and in rats bred in stock colonies an increased salt intake raises the blood pressure. This rise can be partly offset by increased potassium intake. Once high blood pressure is established in these species, lowering the salt intake will not always result in decreased blood pressure.

In human epidemiological studies it was concluded that sodium intake and blood pressure are not always related within any particular community. There is, however, a direct relation between potassium excretion, the sodium/potassium ratio in the urine and blood pressure. The higher the blood level of potassium the lower the blood pressure. In Africa, tribesmen who move from rural areas to the cities develop higher blood pressure that is in part related to an increased salt intake. In one study, where Africans were deliberately given an extra 16g salt in their daily diets, their blood pressure rose. One reason for this effect of salt is that people who have some inherent abnormality in their kidneys cannot excrete the excess sodium.

Prevention of high blood pressure by reducing salt intake has been proved to be effective in animal experiments. No parallel work is available on human beings but babies fed on a low salt diet for the first year of life had lower blood pressure levels than those fed normal salt intakes.

Treatment of high blood pressure by reducing salt intake is effective in some individuals. Very low salt-containing diets were found to reduce high blood pressure before the introduction of diuretics and other drug treatments. Simply halving salt intake to 3.5g (one level teaspoonful) daily can reduce blood pressure by the same amount as that by one tablet of blood pressure-lowering drugs. These drugs are more effective if salt intake is reduced at the same time. The higher the blood pressure the more effective are the drugs on a salt-restricted diet. Those people with only mildly raised blood pressure can sometimes reduce their blood pressure to normal values and maintain it by simple salt restriction.

The positive effect of salt restriction and sodium restriction from other sources is enhanced if the intake of potassium is increased at the same time. It is likely too that adequate intakes of calcium and magnesium are also important in reducing high blood pressure to normal values or in maintaining these values.

Salt retention is also associated with other conditions:

1. Premenstrual oedema. Many women gain weight and experience a bloated feeling a few days before their periods. Symptoms include swelling of the abdomen, ankles and fingers and they are due to retention of water. This oedema can be prevented or reduced by cutting down on the salt intake and at the same time increasing potassium intake by eating more fresh fruit and vegetables and by drinking fresh fruit and vegetable juices.

2. Crash dieting. Fasting or severe calorie-restricted diets that are favoured for rapid weight loss are effective in the short term, but resumption of normal meals after several days can result in sodium retention and hence oedema.

3. Heart failure. When the arteries of the body, including those of the heart, become constricted, the heart works harder to pump out blood and its muscle may become damaged. The kidneys respond by retaining sodium in an attempt to assist the heart but the result is retention of water in many parts of the body including that around the heart. A vicious circle results because the heart works harder when oedema is present, and the usual consequence is heart failure. Diuretic drugs help remove this excess water but their action is improved if salt (i.e. sodium) intake is restricted at the same time.

4. Liver disease. The kidneys may respond to liver damage as they do to heart muscle damage by retaining sodium and hence water. Salt and sodium restriction in the diet can complement conventional medical treatment but the possibility of abnormally low body levels of sodium must be considered.

5. Kidney disease. In some kidney complaints the organ has lost the ability to rid the body of excess salt and high blood pressure results. Some salt and sodium restriction is therefore necessary but the extent of this is the province of the medical practitioner since in severe kidney disease sodium

reduction may exacerbate the condition. In nephrotic syndrome where massive amounts of protein are lost in the urine there is often retention of water and sodium. This is one kidney disease where dietary salt restriction can safely be undertaken in conjunction with diuretic and other drug treatments. Sometimes in rare cases the kidney is unable to retain sodium and excessive quantities are lost in the urine. Here sodium restriction is undesirable and extra salt may have to be eaten; this should only be done under professional advice.

Restricted salt regime is a diet where dietary sodium is reduced to about one-third of normal by eliminating salt added at table; reducing that added during cooking processes to a minimum; selecting foods with low sodium levels. Foods which are rich sources of sodium should be avoided. On this regime the intake of sodium is 2.3g equivalent to 5.9g salt. General guidelines are:

1. no table salt allowed;
2. salt added during cooking and baking powder must be reduced to a minimum;
3. ham, bacon, sausages, tinned meats, tinned fish, shellfish, cheese, sauces, biscuits, scones and shop cakes must not be eaten;
4. bread of any type is restricted to five thin slices per day; butter intake must not exceed 30g (one ounce);
5. meat and fish in small helpings are allowed;
6. sodium-containing vegetables like beetroot, celery, carrots, radish, turnip and watercress are allowed in small quantities as long as no extra salt is added to them. Potatoes cooked in their skins without added salt are allowed;
7. one egg per day is allowed, as is a total of 250ml (half-pint) of milk;
8. intake of fruits and nuts (unsalted) is unlimited;
9. there is no restriction on sugar, honey, jams, rice and sago;
10. salads without added salt are allowed but dressings are not permitted unless they are of the low sodium type.

Low sodium diets are more difficult to organize at home without expert dietary instructions and supervision. One important aspect is that salt-free bread and butter are essential. This is easier when both are home-made but they are available in some shops, as are salt-free polyunsaturated margarines. The sodium intake on the following daily regime is no more than 1.2g equivalent to 3.1g salt.

Daily allowance of milk is 250ml (half-pint), preferably of the low sodium variety; that of low-sodium butter or margarine is 30g (one ounce). *Breakfast:* fruit or fruit juice; low salt cereal; milk from allowance and sugar; one egg (unsalted); low sodium bread or toast; butter from allowance; jam or marmalade; coffee or tea with milk from allowance. *Lunch:* fruit or fruit juice; 90g (3 ounces) unsalted meat, poultry or fresh white fish, either grilled or fried in vegetable oil; potato or rice or pasta; permitted vegetable; salad with low-sodium dressing; low-sodium bread and butter from allowance; fruit sweetened with honey or sugar; tea or coffee with milk from allowance. *Evening meal:* fruit or fruit-juice; 60g (2 ounces) meat or fish or one egg; permitted vegetable and salad with low-sodium dressing; low-sodium bread with butter or margarine from allowance; tea or coffee with milk from allowance. *Bedtime:* remainder of milk allowance.

The following must be avoided: all cured, tinned and pickled meats and fish; canned vegetables and soups; cheeses; bottled sauces; pickled vegetables; sausages; any foods with the ingredients bicarbonate of soda, baking powder, sodium benzoate, monosodium glutamate or any sodium salt listed under sodium-food additives. Potassium chloride may be substituted to flavour some foods but the taste will be found to be different from that when sodium chloride is used.

Savoy cabbage,   good levels of potassium and calcium with significant amounts of phosphorus, sulphur and small quantities of the trace elements. Low sodium food. Figures for mineral levels, when raw and boiled respectively (in mg per 100g) are: sodium 23, 8; potassium 260, 120; calcium 75, 53; magnesium 20, 7; phosphorus 68, 27; iron 0.9, 0.7; copper 0.07, 0.07; zinc 0.3, 0.2; sulphur 88, 30; chloride 22, 9.

---

sea salt,   mainly sodium chloride but contains significant quantities of other salts. A typical composition (in g per 100g) is: sodium chloride 77.82; magnesium chloride 9.44; magnesium sulphate 6.57; calcium sulphate 3.44; potassium chloride 2.11; magnesium bromide 0.22; calcium carbonate trace.

---

seafood,   the crustacea crab, lobster, prawn, scampi and shrimp contain good amounts of calcium, potassium, phosphorus, sulphur and chloride. They are particularly rich in the trace elements iron, copper, zinc and iodine. High sodium levels in most species.

The molluscs cockles, mussels, oysters, scallops, whelks and winkles supply good quantities of sodium, potassium, calcium, phosphorus, sulphur and chloride. They are particularly rich in iron, copper and zinc.

Mineral contents for edible parts of crustacea range (in mg per 100g) from: sodium 120-3840; potassium 100-400; calcium 29-320; magnesium 30-110; phosphorus 150-350; iron 1.3-5.3; copper 0.23-4.8; zinc 0.6-5.3; sulphur 340-510; chloride 530-5850. Shrimps are the richest crustacean source of minerals. Mineral contents for edible parts of molluscs range (in mg per 100g) from: sodium 210-3520; potassium 150-480; calcium 54-200; magnesium 23-360; phosphorus 200-340; iron 3-26; copper 0.28-7.6; zinc 1.2-45; sulphur 250-570; chloride 320-5220. Cockles supply the most iron (can be as high as 40mg per 100g); oysters supply the most zinc (range from 6-100mg per 100g) and the most copper (7.6mg per 100g); whelks and winkles are the richest all-round mollusc sources of minerals. *See also* fish.

---

seakale, moderate but significant quantities of potassium, calcium, phosphorus, sulphur and the trace elements. Iodine content varies over range 20-50µg per 100g. In boiled state provides the following minerals (in mg per 100g); sodium 4; potassium 50; calcium 48; magnesium 11; phosphorus 34; iron 0.6; copper 0.07; sulphur 52; chloride 12.

---

selenium, chemical symbol Se. Atomic weight 79.0. Name derived from the moon goddess Selene. Until 1957, selenium was regarded as a poison, then Dr Klaus Schwartz of the University of California discovered the mineral was essential to prevent liver-tissue degeneration in rats. Now regarded as an essential trace mineral in animals and man.

Irregular distribution of the mineral occurs in the soil of various countries and areas within one country. Low levels in general are contained in Europe, the USA, Australia and New Zealand and high levels in the Far East (Formosa, Japan, Thailand, the Philippines), Puerto Rico, Venezuela and Costa Rica. However, within the UK Norfolk has a selenium-rich soil; in the USA Wyoming and the Dakotas have particularly high soil levels. Epidemiological studies indicate that people who live in areas of low selenium soils may have a prevalence of certain diseases like cancer and heart complaints. In high selenium areas, plants accumulate the mineral, supplying toxic levels to the animals that eat them. 'Blind staggers' and 'alkali disease' are due to toxic intakes of selenium in grazing animals. Those grazing on selenium-deficient soils develop 'white muscle disease' and complaints involving the liver, brain and other organs.

Adult body content of selenium is about 20mg and it is found in all human tissues with the highest concentration in the liver, kidneys and, in the male, the testes. Blood levels vary depending upon the geographical region but in healthy adults average out round 12µg per 100ml. In malnutrition these can drop within the range 8-11µg per 100ml; in well-nourished people from high selenium areas the blood serum level is from 14-22µg per 100ml.

Foods generally contain concentrations of selenium in the following order (in µg per 100g): organ meats 40; fish and shellfish 32; muscle meats 18; wholegrains and cereals 12; dairy products 5; fruit and vegetables 2. Levels in wheat, grain and vegetable crops vary widely depending upon the soil in which they are grown. Similarly milk and eggs as sources of selenium vary considerably according to its soil status — as much as tenfold. Thus milk can contain from 0.5-5µg per 100ml; eggs can supply from 5.6-50µg per 100g. Food processing and refining decrease selenium levels dramatically, e.g. brown rice has 15 times the mineral content of white rice; wholemeal bread contains twice as much as white bread. Brewer's yeast is a rich source; torula yeast contains virtually nil.

Absorption from the food depends on the form of selenium; organically bound it is more efficiently absorbed and assimilated than inorganic. Supplementation of adults with 25µg per day per kg body weight (i.e. supplying a 70kg person with 1750µg) of inorganic selenium (sodium selenite) increased blood levels by only 3.3µg per 100ml. A total of 150µg as selenium yeast increased blood levels by 7.0µg per 100ml. This means that a tenfold lower oral dosage of selenium yeast produced a twofold increase in blood levels of the mineral; the organic form can thus be considered 20 times more effective than the inorganic sodium selenite. Absorption may be uncontrolled but the body is able to assimilate and retain organically bound selenium as in yeast better than the trace mineral in inorganic salts.

Functions of selenium include:
1. preservation of normal liver function;
2. maintenance of the immune defence mechanisms through the white blood cells:
3. protection against toxic minerals such as cadmium and mercury;
4. an essential role in the male reproductive capacity through its high concentration in semen;
5. the production of the essential hormones called prostaglandins;
6. maintenance of normal sight and healthy eyes;
7. maintenance of healthy skin and hair;

8. an anti-inflammatory effect;

9. maintenance of a healthy heart;

10. protection against free radicals, intracellular hydrogen peroxide, and other pollutants by virtue of its presence in the protective enzyme glutathione peroxidase;

11. a protective action against cancer, based on epidemiological evidence;

12. a synergistic action with vitamin E in maintaining the functions of mitochondria, the energy-producing apparatus in all body cells;

13. production of ubiquinone;

14. an anti-oxidant action.

Causes of deficiency include: living exclusively on foods grown in selenium-deficient soils; high intake of processed and refined foods in the diet; feeding babies on formula milks instead of breast milk; solutions used in kidney dialysis that lack the mineral; intravenous feeding solutions.

Deficiency conditions based on animal experiments and human epidemiological studies are: white muscle disease (nutritional muscular dystrophy) in grazing animals characterized by skeletal and heart muscle degeneration; Keshan disease in China, a congestive heart disease; high blood pressure; angina pectoris; muscular pain; arthritis in animals; cancer, particularly of the breast and gastrointestinal tract; infertility in the male; low resistance to infection; infant cot deaths.

Therapy with selenium has been claimed successful in treating the following complaints observed in animals or induced in experimental animals: white muscle disease also known as nutritional muscular dystrophy in lambs; liver disease in rats; infertility in males; low resistance to infection; arthritis; high blood pressure; angina pectoris; Keshan disease (human); cancer; hair, skin and nail problems; ageing effects; detoxification of arsenic, cadmium and mercury; cataract formation; lack of ubiquinone production.

Supplementary forms include selenium-rich yeast; sodium selenite. Supplementary intakes above 200mcg selenium daily (as selenium yeast) are not recommended. Yeast is preferable to selenite as it is less toxic.

Recommended dietary intake is suggested only by the USA governmental authority as follows (in μg per day): infants 0-0.5 year, 10-40; 0.5-1.0 year, 20-60; children 1-3 yrs, 20-80; 4-6 yrs, 30-120; 7-10 yrs, 50-200; 11 + yrs, 50-200; adults, 50-200.

In the USA and Canada intakes have been estimated at between 60 and 224μg selenium daily. In parts of New Zealand daily dietary intakes are as low as 20μg. A daily total intake of between 200 and 300μg selenium is considered by researchers to be the most effective and safe.

Excessive intakes can occur in animals grazing on selenium-rich soil. Signs of chronic toxicity are loss of appetite; loss of weight; muscular weakness; roughened coat; loss of long hair; hoof lesions; malformed offspring. In hens, selenium toxicity causes loss of appetite; reduced growth; decreased egg laying; decreased egg size; lowered or no hatchability; deformed offspring including underdeveloped beak, abnormal development of the feet, legs and neck, fusing of the two outside toes.

In human beings, selenium toxicity from chronic exposure by inhalation and skin contact causes severe irritation of the respiratory tract; severe dermatitis; gastrointestinal disturbances; nausea; nervousness; deformed offspring that have been aborted or born.

Children living in high selenium areas in the USA and parts of Europe have a higher incidence of dental caries. Dietary selenium is incorporated into protein (as selenomethionine) during development and this inhibits mineralization of teeth. Excessive dietary intakes of selenium in man are unusual but accidental overdose has caused hair loss, skin depigmentation, abnormal nails and lassitude. An early sign of excessive intake is a garlicky odour on the breath even when this particular plant has not been eaten. Selenium yeast is less toxic than selenium salts.

Relationship to vitamin E is a potentiation of the effects of either nutrient when in the presence of the other and may be summed up thus:
1.   Selenium can 'spare' vitamin E; the protective action of high potency vitamin E on the heart can be equalled by lower potencies of the vitamin in the presence of the trace mineral.
2.   Selenium is between 50 and 100 times more active as an anti-oxidant than vitamin E.
3.   The protective enzyme glutathione peroxidase requires both selenium and vitamin E to function.
4.   Both nutrients act in the detoxification of harmful free radicals but in this function vitamin E is destroyed and selenium is not.
5.   A combination of selenium with vitamin E gave better relief from angina pectoris than either nutrient alone. In one trial, 92 per cent of patients benefited by reduction of elimination of angina attacks; increased vigour and work capacity; improved electrocardiograms (ECG).
6.   Both nutrients were needed to increase the body's resistance to bacteria and viral infections.
7.   Cancers induced in experimental animals were inhibited by the trace mineral selenium plus the vitamins E and C.
8.   Selenium, vitamins E and C protected against skin cancers induced

by excessive ultraviolet light or excessive sunshine exposure.

---

selenium sulphide, used only as a shampoo in the treatment of dandruff and seborrhoeic dermatitis of the scalp. It is highly toxic if taken internally. If swallowed, the stomach should be emptied by aspiration and lavage and a purgative such as sodium sulphate (30g in 250ml water) given as a solution. Vitamin C, 10mg per kg body weight, given by mouth assists the removal of selenium sulphide through the kidneys.

Hair levels of selenium are increased after the application of shampoos containing selenium sulphide.

---

selenium yeast, provides up to $1000\mu g$ selenium per gram of yeast. Produced by adding inorganic selenium salts to growing yeast which incorporates the trace mineral into its protein. This involves replacement of the sulphur in the sulphur-containing amino acids by selenium. The main protein constituent is selenomethionine. Selenium in yeast protein is better absorbed, better utilized and less toxic than inorganic selenium salts.

---

sherry, low in sodium but supplies moderate quantities of potassium and iron with small amounts of all other minerals. It contains the following quantities, for dry, medium and sweet variety respectively (in mg per 100g): sodium 10, 6, 13; potassium 57, 89, 110; calcium 7, 9, 7; magnesium 13, 8, 11; phosphorus 11, 7, 10; iron 0.39, 0.53, 0.37; copper 0.03, 0.10, 0.11; zinc 0.27 for medium variety; chloride 12, 7, 14.

---

silica gel, provides 46.8mg silicon in 100mg gel. Used in tabletting as a suspending, disintegrating and anti-cooking agent. Usually up to 10mg of silica gel per tablet.

---

silicon, chemical symbol Si. Atomic weight 28.1. Found in nature as silica (silicon oxide) in quartz, sand, sandstone; as silicates in feldspar, kaolinate, anorthite. The second most abundant element on earth (next to oxygen), constituting about 27.6g per 100g in the earth's crust.

Silicon and silicon salts are so insoluble that only trace amounts are found in body tissues. It has been shown to be an essential trace element for the growing rat and chick; deficiency in these species leads to abnormalities in the bones. In addition, it is an essential component of cartilage where it is important for the strength and elasticity of the gristle. Silicon helps keep arterial walls elastic, an important feature of blood pressure control. All connective tissue of the body contains silicon. All studies have been carried out on animals but similar functions probably apply to human beings also.

Toxic effects of silicon are confined to the inhalation of silica as dust from coal, glass manufacture, ceramics production and sand-blasting of rocks. The resulting disease is silicosis where particles of silica are deposited in the lungs, setting up irritation and eventually loss of elasticity.

Silicon compounds used in tabletting include silicon dioxide.

---

silicon dioxide, also known as silica, colloidal silica. Provides 46.8mg silicon in 100mg. Used in the same way as silica gel (see entry).

---

silver, a food additive used as a surface colouring agent; E174. Chemical symbol Ag from the Latin *argentum*. Atomic weight 108. Acceptable daily intake not determined. Permitted only on dragées and on sugar-coated flour confectionery.

---

sodium, chemical symbol Na, from the Latin *natrium*. Atomic weight 23.0. An alkali metal that occurs naturally as sodium chloride, sodium bromide, sodium silicates and sodium carbonates. Abundance in earth's crust is 2.8 per cent.

Adult body content (65kg weight) of sodium in a healthy individual is about 92g, equivalent to 234g sodium chloride. More than half the sodium is in the fluids that bathe the cells (extracellular); 34.5g is present in the bones; less than 11.5g is retained within the cells (intracellular). Bone sodium is not generally available as an immediate reserve since it is enmeshed in the crystals of the insoluble bone minerals. If sodium is injected into the body as common salt, it quickly equilibrates with both intracellular and extracellular sodium, but exchange with bone sodium is almost negligible. The total exchangeable sodium in the body is therefore about 64.4g and it is this sodium that changes rapidly, depending upon its intake from the diet and the excretion of the mineral.

Daily intakes of sodium from the food are from 1.61-6.90g which corresponds to 4.10-17.55g common salt. The food as eaten contributes only 4.6g sodium daily (corresponding to 11.7g common salt), the remainder being added as table salt.

In babies, the ideal sodium content of food is that of human breast milk (180mg per litre). Unmodified cow's milk contains 770mg per litre so it should not be fed to babies in the first three months of life. Animal experiments indicate that too much salt in a baby's diet can cause high blood pressure and even death. UK and USA health authorities recommend that salt should not be added during the processing and preparation of infant foods.

Foods as they occur in nature do not generally have high amounts of sodium but the mineral is added in large amounts as sodium chloride (common salt) during cooking, refining, processing and preservation of foods or as sodium bicarbonate in baking powder or as monosodium glutamate. Bakers, for example, add salt to bread at a level of about 1 per cent; butter, bacon, processed meats, tinned foods in general are all salted in preparation. An ordinary diet without salt supplementation in this way will provide ample sodium for body needs; added salt at the table is simply an acquired taste.

Rich sources of sodium are (in mg per 100g): yeast extract 4640; bacon 1900; smoked fish 1000-1800; salami 1800; sauces 1100-1400; cornflakes 1200; canned or boiled ham 1200; savoury biscuits 610-1200; processed cheese and cheese spread 1360; Danish Blue cheese 1420; Camembert cheese 1410; Stilton cheese 1150; corned beef 910; Edam cheese 980; salted butter 870; margarine 800; sausage 780; Cheddar and other hard cheeses 610; cottage cheese 450; bread 560; fresh and tinned shellfish 210-550; tinned vegetables 230-330.

Moderate sources of sodium are (in mg per 100g): sweet biscuits 200-500; self-raising flour 350; cream cheese 300; root vegetables 60-140; eggs 140; fresh fish 100; raw meats 60-90; yogurt 64-76; pulses 30-60; cornflour 52; oatmeal 33; single cream 42; dried fruits 30.

Poor sources of sodium are (in mg per 100g): fresh fruit 1-30; unsalted nuts 1-20; green vegetables 2-13; fruit juices 1-4; rice 6; flour 2-4; sago 3; lard 2. For other levels see individual foods.

Foods of animal and fish origin usually contain more sodium than wholegrains, fruits, vegetables, unsalted nuts and fruits. Poultry supply only moderate amounts.

Absorption of sodium as common salt or in any soluble form from the intestines is passive so excessive intakes are as easily absorbed as moderate ones. There is no control of absorption as with most other minerals so the gastrointestinal tract plays little part in controlling body levels.

Excretion of sodium is mainly via the kidneys and the resulting urine usually contains from 920-2300mg sodium per litre. Increased intake of the mineral leads to increased excretion and normal healthy kidneys have no difficulty in excreting the excess as long as there is sufficient water excreted. There is a limit to the amount by which the kidneys can concentrate urine (specific gravity of about 1.035 is the maximum), so high intakes of sodium, usually as salt, must be accompanied by large volumes of water. Excessive salt intakes usually induce thirst which when slaked compensates for the increased requirements of water. The highest excretion of sodium occurs about midday, with the lowest at night.

Control of urinary excretion of sodium is under the influence of hormones. These act upon the kidney tubules by stimulating or slowing the reabsorption of sodium within the kidney. One hormone is aldosterone which is elaborated in the adrenal cortex. When the body sodium is depleted, e.g. by excessive sweating or by starvation, aldosterone is secreted and this stimulates the kidney to reabsorb and hence conserve the sodium in the urine. In Addison's disease, aldosterone is no longer produced because the adrenal cortex is destroyed and sodium is excreted in large, uncontrolled amounts. The result is muscular weakness and low blood pressure. Treatment is to give sufficient sodium in the form of salt to replace the losses and to supply the hormone by injection. Diseased kidneys as in renal failure are unable to conserve sodium and the individual becomes markedly depleted.

Excessive amounts of aldosterone and other adrenal cortex hormones will cause increased retention of sodium. This also happens in congestive heart disease and in certain types of kidney disease. The usual result is high blood pressure.

Faecal excretion of sodium is very small, usually only about 115mg daily. All the digestive juices contain large amounts of sodium but most of this is reabsorbed in the large intestine. In diarrhoea, reabsorption is inefficient and significant daily losses of sodium up to 2070mg are possible in the faeces. These must be replaced in chronic diarrhoea to prevent body depletion.

Excretion through the skin is usually negligible, but when sweating is excessive losses can be significant. Sweat contains from 460-1840mg sodium per litre but in those who are acclimatized to heat this is maintained at 960mg per litre. In tropical climates or whilst indulging in heavy manual work excretion of sweat can reach up to 14 litres so sodium loss then becomes serious and more significant than urinary loss. Without supplementary salt in these conditions, sodium depletion soon follows. Miner's cramp is one such condition.

Sodium balance in a healthy individual should be zero. For example, with a good intake of 3105mg and no salt added at table, excretion should be 2990mg in the urine plus 115mg in the faeces; sweat excretion is negligible if the individual is sedentary. Under conditions of hard exercise or manual work sweating can induce a negative balance, i.e. more sodium is excreted than eaten. Excessive intakes and certain diseases can cause positive balance where the extra sodium in the diet is not excreted. Negative balance is usually treated by increased oral intake of sodium; positive balance by diuretic drugs.

Deficiency of sodium is highly unlikely on any diet but it can be associated with dehydration as in heat exhaustion brought on by high temperatures, hard exercise, manual work; in babies it can be caused by diarrhoea. The extracellular fluid volume is reduced, as is the blood volume. The blood thickens, veins collapse, blood pressure is reduced and the pulse becomes rapid. These changes cause dryness of the mouth even though thirst may be absent. There is usually mental apathy, loss of appetite and sometimes vomiting. Muscle cramps are usually present. Dehydration is also indicated by sunken features — particularly the eyes, which recede — and a loose, non-elastic skin.

Deficiency of sodium may occur without water depletion; the condition is called water intoxication. It occurs after heavy sweating when the thirst is quenched with water to which no sodium has been added; in the treatment of sodium deficiency if too much water is given by mouth or intravenously; in the treatment of dehydration if only water is given. Symptoms include loss of appetite; weakness; mental apathy; muscular twitchings; convulsions; coma induced by excessive retention of water by the brain. Treatment is to ensure that salt is added to replacement fluids in the above conditions.

Causes of low blood sodium levels may also be due to kidney failure; hormonal imbalance, e.g. excess production of anti-diuretic hormone or vasopressin; lung cancers; lung infections; meningitis; myxoedema; lack of adrenal and pituitary hormones; oedema as in heart failure, liver cirrhosis, nephrotic syndrome, nephritis, toxaemia of pregnancy; high blood glucose levels; porphyria. Treatment of low blood sodium in these conditions is salt replacement, hormones and successful correction of the underlying disease.

Excess of sodium in the body accumulates primarily in the extracellular fluids. As the concentration rises the body responds by passing more water into the extracellular fluids to dilute out the sodium so oedema results. Consequences of high salt intake that is not excreted are therefore high blood pressure; enlarged heart; abnormal ECG tracings; enlarged kidneys, leading to nephritis. Epidemiological evidence shows that high blood pressure in some countries is associated with habitual high salt intakes. Elevation of blood serum sodium concentration is indicative of a deficit in body water relative to sodium.

Causes of high blood sodium levels include diabetes insipidus where vasopressin is deficient; kidney failure; high blood calcium; low blood potassium; excessive sweating without access to water, e.g. infants, bedridden or comatose patients; excessive diarrhoea, especially in children; grossly excessive intakes of sodium with limited access to water. Treatment is water replacement usually accompanied by drug diuretic treatment; restriction of sodium in the diet; occasionally kidney dialysis.

Functions of sodium are:
1. in maintaining a normal balance of water between body cells and the surrounding fluids. Potassium also contributes to this.
2. in nerve impulse transmission where the flow of sodium into the nerve cell and the opposite flow of potassium out of the cell sets up an electrical impulse that travels down the nerve to the muscle;
3. in all muscle contraction including that of the heart where the correct balance of sodium and potassium is essential for a smooth response;
4. in preserving the acid-alkali balance of the body in close relationship with bicarbonate, phosphate and protein and the minerals potassium, calcium and magnesium;
5. as a constituent of ATPase, the enzyme responsible for splitting adenosine triphosphate in the production of energy;
6. the active transport of the nutrients amino acids and glucose into body cells.

Supplementary form of sodium is sodium chloride which provides 39.3mg sodium in 100mg chloride.

Recommended daily intake has not been suggested by any authority since insufficiency in the diet is highly unlikely.

Food additives of sodium, apart from those found in natural foods, include sodium acetate; sodium alginate; sodium aluminium phosphate, acidic and basic; sodium ascorbate; sodium benzoate; sodium biphenyl-2-yl oxide; sodium bicarbonate; sodium carbonate; sodium caseinate; sodium chloride; sodium hydrogen citrate; trisodium citrate; tetrasodium diphosphate; trisodium diphosphate; sodium ferrocyanide; sodium gluconate; sodium heptonate; sodium dihydrogen citrate; sodium hydrogen diacetate; disodium dihydrogen diphosphate; disodium dihydrogen ethylenediamine — NNN'N'-tetra-acetate; sodium hydrogen glutamate (monosodium glutamate); sodium hydrogen malate; sodium dihydrogen orthophosphate; disodium hydrogen orthophosphate; sodium hydrogen sulphite; sodium hydroxide; sodium lactate; sodium malate; sodium metabisulphite; sodium nitrate; sodium nitrite; trisodium orthophosphate; sodium pectate; sodium polyphosphates; sodium propionate; sodium 5'-ribonucleotide; soaps or sodium salts of fatty acids; sodium sesquicarbonate; sodium sorbate; sodium stearoyl-2-lactate; sodium sulphate; sodium sulphite; disodium tartrates; monosodium tartrates; pentasodium triphosphate; sodium potassium tartrate; sodium hydrogen malate.

Drugs containing sodium include sodium alginate, sodium bicarbonate — antacids; sodium acetate and sodium lactate — metabolic acidosis; sodium phosphate, sodium sulphate and sodium tartrate — purgatives; sodium ascorbate — vitamin; sodium calcium edetate — treatment of heavy metal poisoning; sodium carboxymethylcellulose — bulking and swelling agent; sodium citrate — cough mixtures; sodium cromoglycate — asthma; sodium fusidate — corticosteroid; sodium hyaluronate — eye preparation; sodium lauryl sulphate — laxative; sodium lauryl sulphoacetate — laxative; sodium nitroprusside — angina treatment; sodium oleate — haemorrhoid treatment; sodium perborate — gingivitis; sodium picosulphate — laxative; sodium pyrrolidone carboxylate — skin cleanser; sodium ricinoleate — gingivitis; sodium saccharin — sweetener; sodium salicylate — asthma; sodium valproate — epilepsy.

---

sodium acetate, a food additive used as a buffer. Acceptable daily intake is not limited. Provides 28.0mg sodium per 100mg. Permitted as a miscellaneous additive.

---

sodium acid phosphate, also known as sodium dihydrogen phosphate; sodium biphosphate; monosodium orthophosphate; sodium dihydrogen orthophosphate dihydrate. Provides 14.7mg sodium and 19.9mg phosphorus in 100mg phosphate. Has been given with sodium phosphate in the treatment of hypercalcaemia (too much calcium in the blood). Given by mouth to make the urine more acid. It is poorly absorbed from the gastrointestinal system and retains water within the intestine acting as a mild purgative, evacuating the bowel in 1-2 hrs. Used rectally as an enema. When added to pre-sweetened breakfast cereal at 1 per cent level it reduces the incidence of dental caries in children. Therapeutic dose is 2-4g phosphate as required.

sodium alginate, a food additive used as an emulsifier or stabilizer; as a gelling agent; as a boiler water additive; E401. Acceptable daily intake is up to 50mg per kg body weight. Provides very small amounts of sodium. Permitted in whipping cream for caterers or food manufacturers; as a diluent for food colours; in boiler feed water for direct steam treatment of milk; in certain cheeses, as an emulsifier or stabilizer; in reduced-sugar jam products.

sodium aluminate, a food additive that is used as a boiler feed water additive for direct steam treatment of milk. Provides 28mg sodium and 32.9mg aluminium per 100mg.

sodium aluminium phosphate, acidic, a food additive used as an acid; as a raising agent for flour. Acceptable daily intake up to 254mg per kg body weight at normal calcium intakes. Provides 7.7mg sodium, 6.0mg aluminium and 27.6mg phosphorus per 100mg. Permitted miscellaneous additive.

sodium aluminium phosphate, basic, a food additive used as an emulsifying salt. Acceptable daily intake up to 250mg per kg body weight at normal calcium intakes. Provides 28.3mg sodium, 8.3mg aluminium and 19.1mg phosphorus per 100mg. Permitted miscellaneous additive.

sodium ascorbate, a food additive used as an antioxidant; as a colour preservative; as vitamin C; E301. Acceptable daily intake not specified. Provides 11.6mg sodium per 100mg. Permitted as antioxidant; in dried-milk products. Prohibited in unprocessed meats.

sodium benzoate, a food additive used as a preservative, E211.

Acceptable daily intake up to 5mg per kg body weight. Provides 16.0mg sodium per 100mg. Permitted only in certain foods, quantity restricted.

---

sodium bicarbonate, also known as sodium hydrogen carbonate. A food additive used as an alkali; as an aerating agent; as a diluent. Acceptable daily intake not limited. Provides 27.4mg sodium per 100mg. Permitted in soda bread; in soda water; in certain types of cream; as a diluent for food colours; in certain cocoa products; in condensed-milk and dried-milk products; in jams and similar products; as a miscellaneous additive.

---

sodium diphenyl-2-yl oxide, a food additive used as a preservative. Also known as sodium orthophenylphenate; E232. Provides 12.0mg sodium per 100mg. Permitted in citrus fruits, quantity restricted.

---

sodium bisulphite, also known as sodium hydrogen sulphite; acid sodium sulphite. A food additive that functions as a preservative, E222. Acceptable daily intake is up to 0.7mg per kg body weight. Provides 22.1mg sodium and 30.8mg sulphur per 100mg. Permitted in most specified sugar products; in some fruit juices; in certain other foods.

---

sodium carbonate, a food additive used as an alkali. Acceptable daily intake not limited. Provides 43.4mg sodium per 100mg. Permitted in sterilized or UHT cream; as a diluent for food colours; in certain cocoa products; in boiler feed water for direct steam treatment of milk; in jams and similar products; as a miscellaneous additive.

---

sodium caseinate, a food additive used as an emulsifier or stabilizer; as a dietary source of protein. Acceptable daily intake is not limited. Provides very small amount of sodium. Permitted in all foods.

---

sodium diacetate, also known as sodium hydrogen diacetate. A food additive used as a buffer; as a preservative; E262. Acceptable daily intake up to 15mg per kg body weight. Provides 16.2mg sodium per 100mg. Permitted in bread; as a miscellaneous additive.

---

sodium dihydrogen citrate, also known as monosodium citrate. A food additive used as a buffer; as an emulsifying salt; as a sequestrant; E331. Acceptable daily intake not limited. Provides 6.9mg sodium per 100mg. Permitted in sterilized and UHT cream; in some cheeses; in condensed-milk and dried-milk products; in jam and similar products (for controlling acidity only); as a miscellaneous additive.

sodium diphosphate, dibasic, a food additive also known as disodium hydrogen orthophosphate. A food additive that functions as a buffer; as a gelling agent; as a stabilizer; as a nutrient; E339. Acceptable daily intake up to 350mg per kg body weight. Provides 32.4mg sodium and 21.8mg phosphorus per 100mg. Permitted in sterilized and UHT cream; in some cheeses; in condensed-milk and dried-milk products; in boiler feed water for direct steam treatment of milk; as a miscellaneous additive.

sodium ferrocyanide, also known as sodium hexacyanoferrate II. Used as a food additive, functioning as an anti-caking agent; as a crystal modifier. Acceptable daily intake up to 0.025mg per kg body weight. Provides 19.0mg sodium and 11.6mg iron per 100mg. Permitted as a miscellaneous additive.

sodium fluoride, provides 45.2mg fluoride and 54.8mg sodium in 100mg. Used for the fluoridation of drinking water in amounts sufficient to make the final concentration of fluoride 1mg per litre. Prophylactic dose to prevent dental caries is 2.2mg daily (contains 1mg fluoride). Used also in dental gels for direct application to teeth. Present in mouth rinses for preventing dental caries at a strength of 2g per 100ml; in paediatric drops at a potency of 1.1mg in each 10-drop dose; in tablets, each containing 2.2mg; in toothpastes.

Recommended doses of sodium fluoride should not be exceeded as it is a toxic substance. Taken by mouth in quantities more than 250mg it causes salivation; nausea; vomiting; pain above the stomach; diarrhoea. Larger quantities cause muscular weakness; convulsions; respiratory and heart failure and death within 2-4 hrs. Other effects of chronic intake of slightly toxic levels include acne; hypothyroidism; hypersensitivity; skeletal fluorosis.

sodium gluconate, a food additive used as a sequestrant; as a source of sodium in dietary supplements. Acceptable daily intake up to 50mg per kg body weight. Provides 10.6mg sodium per 100mg. Permitted miscellaneous additive.

sodium glycerophosphate, has been used in the past as source of phosphorus. Provides 9.8mg phosphorus and 14.6mg sodium in 100mg glycerophosphate. Dose is usually 300-600mg up to a daily intake of 4g. Used mainly as a tonic.

sodium heptonate, a food additive used as a sequestrant. Acceptable daily intake not specified. Provides 81.0mg sodium per 100mg. Permitted as a miscellaneous additive.

sodium hydrogen malate, a food additive used as a buffer. Acceptable daily intake not specified. Provides 14.7mg sodium per 100mg. Permitted in jam and similar products; as a miscellaneous additive.

sodium hydroxide, also known as caustic soda. A food additive used as an alkali; as a colour solvent. Acceptable daily intake not limited. Provides 57.5mg sodium per 100mg. Permitted in certain cocoa products; as a diluent for food colours; in boiler feed water for direct steam treatment of milk; in jam and similar products; as a miscellaneous additive.

sodium 5'-inosinate, also known as inosine 5'-(disodium phosphate); disodium inosine 5'-monophosphate. A food additive used as a flavour enhancer. Provides 9.5mg sodium per 100mg. Acceptable daily intake is not specified. Permitted as a miscellaneous additive. Prohibited in foods made for babies and young children.

sodium iodide, provides 84.7µg iodine in 100µg iodide. Used in a similar manner to potassium iodide. Daily dose in pre-operative treatment of thyrotoxicosis is 150mg; as an expectorant 250-500mg. As a supplement 200-1200µg daily. Used to iodize table salt at a level of 10mg per 100g of salt.

sodium lactate, a food additive used as a buffer; as a humectant; as an antioxidant synergist; E325. Acceptable daily intake not limited. Provides 20.5mg sodium per 100mg. Permitted in jam and similar products for normalizing acidity; as a miscellaneous additive.

sodium malate, a food additive used as a buffer. Acceptable daily intake not limited. Provides 25.8mg sodium per 100mg. Permitted in jam and similar products; as a miscellaneous additive.

sodium metabisulphite, a food additive used as a preservative, E223. Acceptable daily intake up to 0.7mg per kg body weight. Provides 24.2mg sodium and 33.7mg sulphur per 100mg. Permitted in most specified sugar products; in some fruit juices; in certain foods, quantity restricted.

sodium metasilicate, a food additive used in water treatment; as a boiler water additive. Provides 37.7mg sodium and 23.0mg silica per 100mg. Permitted in boiler feed water for direct steam treatment of milk.

sodium methyl p-hydroxybenzoate, a food additive that functions as a preservative, E219. Provides 13.2mg sodium per 100mg. Permitted in certain foods but quantity restricted.

sodium molybdate, provides 46.5μg molybdenum and 21.7μg sodium in 100μg molybdate. Daily intake of sodium molybdate should not exceed 0.5mg when used as a supplement as the substance is toxic in large quantities.

sodium monofluorophosphate, provides 13.2mg fluoride in 100mg. Used at a strength of 0.76 per cent in fluoride toothpastes.

sodium nitrate, also known as saltpetre. A food additive used as a preservative; as a curing salt; E251. Acceptable daily intake up to 5mg per kg body weight. Provides 27.1mg sodium per 100mg. Permitted in cured meats; in some cheeses, quantity restricted. May not be added to foods specially made for babies and young children.

---

sodium nitrite,   a food additive used as a preservative; as a curing salt; E250. Acceptable daily intake up to 0.2mg per kg body weight. Provides 33.3mg per 100mg. Permitted in cured meats; in some cheeses. May not be added to food specially prepared for babies and young children.

---

sodium pectate,   a food additive used as an emulsifier or stabilizer; as a gelling agent; E440a. Acceptable daily intake has not been specified. Provides only small amounts of sodium. Permitted as an emulsifier; as a stabilizer; in certain jam products, quantity restricted.

---

sodium phosphate,   also known as disodium hydrogen phosphate; dibasic sodium phosphate; disodium hydrogen orthophosphate dodecahydrate. Provides 12.9mg sodium and 8.7mg phosphorus in 100mg phosphate. Has been used with sodium acid phosphate in the treatment of hypercalcaemia (high level of blood calcium); in treatment of calcium and phosphorus metabolic disorders; in dilute solution it is used as a mild purgative producing a watery evacuation of the bowel within 1-2 hrs. It has a mild diuretic action and renders the urine less acid. Therapeutic dose is 2-16g as required.

---

sodium phosphate, monobasic,   also known as sodium dihydrogen orthophosphate. A food additive used as a buffer, E339. Acceptable daily intake up to 350mg per kg body weight. Provides 19.2mg sodium and 25.8mg phosphorus per 100mg. Permitted in sterilized and UHT cream; in some cheeses; in condensed-milk and dried-milk products; in boiler feed water for direct steam treatment of milk; as a miscellaneous additive.

---

sodium polyphosphates,   also known as sodium hexametaphosphate; sodium tripolyphosphate; tetrasodium pyrophosphate. Food additives used as emulsifying salts; as sequestrants; as stabilizers; E450c. Acceptable daily intake up to 350mg per kg body weight. Provides 31.3mg sodium and 25.3mg phosphorus per 100mg. Permitted in some cheeses; in unsweetened condensed-milk products; in boiler feed water for direct steam treatment of milk; in reduced-sugar jam products; as a miscellaneous additive.

---

sodium propionate,   a food additive that is used as a preservative, E281. Acceptable daily intake not limited. Provides 24.0mg sodium per 100mg. Permitted in bread; flour confectionery; Christmas puddings, quantity restricted.

---

sodium pump,   the mechanism whereby potassium levels inside body cells and sodium levels outside them are kept constant. Cells' membranes are permeable to both minerals when in solution; the concentration gradients are such that potassium tends to flow out of cells and sodium flows in. To maintain the balance of high levels of potassium inside and sodium outside the cells energy is required which is provided by splitting of high-energy phosphate bonds of adenosine triphosphate. The minerals are transported on the backs of glucose and some unknown carrier. Certain factors can affect the efficiency of the sodium pump causing it to slow down. One is ouabain, a plant drug that acts like digitalis; the other is phlorizin, the toxic principle of apple, pear, plum and cherry trees (but not their fruits). Vasopressin, the sodium-excreting hormone from the adrenals, slows down the sodium pump. This increases the blood pressure and it has been shown recently that the sodium pump is slower in those people with high blood pressure.

---

sodium 5'-ribonucleotide,   a food additive used as a flavour enhancer. Acceptable daily intake not specified. Provides very small amounts of sodium. Permitted miscellaneous additive. Prohibited in foods specially made for babies and young children.

---

sodium saccharin,   a food additive, also known as soluble saccharin, used as an artificial sweetener (500 times sweeter than sugar). Acceptable daily intake up to 2.5mg per kg body weight. Provides 9.5mg sodium per 100mg. Permitted in soft drinks; in reduced-sugar and diabetic jam products; as an artificial sweetener. Prohibited in ice-cream.

---

sodium selenite, provides 45.7μg selenium in 100μg selenite. An inorganic selenium salt that has been used to supply selenium to animal feeds or as an addition to selenium-deficient soils. Lethal dose in rats is 70mg per kg body weight. Sometimes used as a food supplement but largely superseded by selenium-yeast. From 90-95 per cent of a 1mg dose of sodium selenite in water is absorbed in human beings.

sodium sesquicarbonate, a food additive used as an alkali. Acceptable daily intake not specified. Provides 30.5mg sodium per 100mg. Permitted as a miscellaneous additive; in certain cocoa products, quantity restricted.

sodium silicofluoride, provides 60.6mg fluoride and 24.4mg sodium in 100mg. Used to fluoridate drinking water.

sodium soaps, food additives used as emulsifiers; as stabilizers; E470. Acceptable daily intake not limited. Provides about 8.0mg sodium per 100mg. Permitted in malted barley; in Dutch rusks; as emulsifiers and stabilizers.

sodium sorbate, a food additive used as a preservative, E201. Acceptable daily intake up to 25mg per kg body weight. Provides 17.2mg sodium per 100mg. Permitted in certain foods, quantity restricted.

sodium stearoyl-2-lactylate, a food additive used as an emulsifier or stabilizer, E481. Acceptable daily intake up to 20mg per kg body weight. Provides only small amounts of sodium. Permitted in bread up to 5g per kg; as an emulsifier or stabilizer.

sodium sulphate, a food additive used as a diluent for food colours. Provides 32.4mg sodium per 100mg. Permitted as a diluent for food colours; in boiler feed water for direct steam treatment of milk; as a miscellaneous additive.

sodium sulphite, a food additive used as a preservative, E221. Acceptable daily intake up to 0.7mg per kg body weight. Provides 36.5mg sodium per 100mg. Permitted in most specified sugar products; in some fruit juices; in boiler feed water for direct steam treatment of milk; as a preservative in certain foods, quantity restricted.

---

sodium tartrate, a food additive used as a buffer; as an emulsifying salt; as a sequestrant; E335. Acceptable daily intake up to 30mg per kg body weight. Provides 12.1mg sodium per 100mg. Permitted in some cheeses; in jam and similar products; as a miscellaneous additive.

---

soluble iron pyrophosphate, provides 10mg iron in 100mg plus 8.3mg phosphorus. Used in a daily dose of 120-500mg pyrophosphate sometimes with cod liver oil emulsions. Widely used in animals, particularly for the prevention of piglet anaemia.

---

soups, all provide high sodium levels (except specific low sodium varieties) but are good sources of potassium, calcium, magnesium, phosphorus, chloride and the trace elements depending upon type.

All figures refer to mineral levels of canned, condensed as eaten and dried as eaten in the following ranges (in mg per 100g): sodium 350-6120; potassium 16-920; calcium 3-140; magnesium 3-48; phosphorus 10-260; iron 0.2-4.3; copper 0.02-0.33; zinc 0.1-2.4; chloride 290-9030.

---

soya flour, devoid of sodium but very rich in potassium, calcium, magnesium and phosphorus. Excellent source of iron.

Full fat supplies (in mg per 100g): sodium 1; potassium 1660; calcium 210; magnesium 240; phosphorus 600; iron 6.9. *Low fat* supplies (in mg per 100g): sodium 1; potassium 2030; calcium 240; magnesium 290; phosphorus 640; iron 9.1.

---

spaghetti, pasta made from wheat flour. Supplies small amounts of all minerals. High sodium and chloride content in canned variety because of added salt. Figures given are for boiled and canned in tomato sauce respectively (in mg per 100g): sodium 2, 500; potassium 50, 130; calcium

7, 21; magnesium 11, 11; phosphorus 37, 30; iron 0.4, 0.4; copper 0.08, 0.13; zinc 0.3 for boiled variety; sulphur 30 in boiled state; chloride 20, 800.

---

spinach, excellent source of calcium, potassium and iron. Provides good intakes of magnesium, phosphorus and sulphur plus the trace elements. Moderate sodium level. As boiled it provides the following mineral levels (in mg per 100g): sodium 120; potassium 490; calcium 600; magnesium 59; phosphorus 93; iron 4.0; copper 0.26; zinc 0.4; sulphur 86; chloride 56.

---

spirulina, a blue-green alga that was used as a staple food by the Aztecs of Mexico and is now being developed as a high-protein food providing significant amounts of minerals. Range of mineral contents of dried material (in mg per 100g) is: calcium 104.5-131.5; magnesium 141.0-191.5; phosphorus 761.7-894.2; iron 47.5-58.0; sodium 27.5-41.2; potassium 1331-1540; chloride 400-440; manganese 1.8-2.5; zinc 2.7-3.9. There are also traces of bismuth, chromium, cobalt and selenium.

---

split dried peas, low sodium food that supplies very good levels of potassium, magnesium, phosphorus and sulphur. Rich source of trace elements. Mineral levels for raw and boiled respectively (in mg per 100g) are: sodium 38, 14; potassium 910, 270; calcium 33, 11; magnesium 130, 30; phosphorus 270, 120; iron 5.4, 1.7; copper 0.58, 0.25; zinc 4.0, 1.2; sulphur 170, 46; chloride 56, 10.

---

spring cabbage, low sodium food with good potassium content and small amounts of the other minerals. When boiled it provides (in mg per 100g): sodium 12; potassium 110; calcium 30; magnesium 6; phosphorus 32; iron 0.5; copper 0.07; zinc 0.2; sulphur 27; chloride 6.

---

spring greens, good source of iron, potassium and calcium with low sodium level. Useful source of other minerals. As boiled it supplies (in mg per 100g): sodium 10; potassium 120; calcium 86; magnesium 9; phosphorus 31; iron 1.3; copper 0.08; zinc 0.4; sulphur 29; chloride 16.

---

spring onions, low sodium food with excellent levels of potassium, calcium and iron. Useful quantities of other minerals also. In the raw state it supplies (in mg per 100g): sodium 13; potassium 230; calcium 140; magnesium 11; phosphorus 24; iron 1.3; copper 0.13; sulphur 50; chloride 36.

---

stannous fluoride, tin fluoride, provides 75.8μg tin and 24.2μg fluoride in 100μg. Used as a fluoride gel directly applied to the teeth to prevent dental caries. Added also to fluoride toothpastes but may stain the teeth.

---

strawberries, main attributes are as good provider of potassium and very low sodium levels. Useful source of trace minerals and others. Mineral levels for raw and canned variety respectively (in mg per 100g) are: sodium 2, 7; potassium 160, 97; calcium 22, 14; magnesium 12, 7; phosphorus 23, 15; iron 0.7, 0.9; copper 0.13, 0.03; zinc 0.1, 0.2; sulphur, raw state provides 13; chloride 18, 5.

---

strontium, named from its discovery in the ore from the lead mines of Strontian in Scotland. Chemical symbol Sr. Atomic weight 87.6. An alkaline earth metal.

No evidence that it is essential for animal and human life. It behaves as calcium and accompanies it in foods rich in calcium, e.g. milk, grains, fresh vegetables. Dietary strontium, like calcium, is concentrated in the bones. The quantity of strontium in biological material is usually about one-thousandth that of calcium.

Cow's milk is richer in both strontium and calcium than human milk. Bottle-fed babies tend to receive intakes of strontium some four times greater than those breast-fed. Some of it is retained. Breast-fed babies excrete more than they receive because their urinary volume is increased. In all babies, the ratio strontium to calcium is higher in the urine and faeces than in the bones. These results suggest that in infants at least the body discriminates against strontium in favour of calcium.

Some epidemiological evidence shows that strontium may have a protective effect against dental caries. One study suggests it may be helpful in the treatment of osteoporosis. It may also protect the energy-producing apparatus of body cells.

---

strontium-90, radioactive form of strontium produced by the effect of nuclear explosions. It can be dispersed over wide areas and so finds its way into plants and thence into animals and man. Like calcium it accumulates in the bones where it can continue to radiate radioactivity. With a half-life of 28 years such effects can eventually become dangerous. Strontium-90 represents the only toxic form of strontium. The non-radioactive mineral appears to be perfectly safe.

---

suet, as sold, provides small amounts of all minerals. As a pudding provides high sodium, calcium and phosphorus intakes with useful quantities of the other elements.

In block and shredded form it provides the following minerals (in mg per 100g): sodium 21, trace; potassium 13, trace; calcium 6, trace; magnesium 1, trace; phosphorus 7, trace; iron 0.4, trace; copper 0.04, trace; zinc, trace found in shredded; sulphur 20, trace; chloride 18, trace.

Suet pudding, steamed, supplies (in mg per 100g): sodium 470; potassium 91; calcium 240; magnesium 14; phosphorus 180; iron 0.9; copper 0.08; zinc 0.4; chloride 510.

---

sugar, demerara type provides significant quantities of all minerals; white variety is practically devoid of minerals. Demerara and white varieties respectively, provide (in mg per 100g): sodium 6, trace; potassium 89, 2; calcium 53, 2; magnesium 15, trace; phosphorus 20, trace; iron 0.9, trace; copper 0.06, 0.02; sulphur 14, trace; chloride 35, trace.

---

sulphur, chemical symbol S. Atomic weight 32.1. Occurs in nature in the free state and in combination as sulphates and sulphides. Constitutes 0.05 per cent of the earth's crust.

As it is a constituent of all proteins it is an essential element for man, animals, plants and micro-organisms. Sulphur content of an adult body is about 100g. The greater part occurs in the three amino acids, cysteine, cystine and methionine. Some is present in the amino acid taurine. The rest appears as sulphate within body cells, either free or attached to body constituents like the anti-blood clotting substance heparin and the structural component chondroitin sulphate.

Sulphur is also present in the two vitamins thiamine and biotin; in vitamin D of milk where it occurs as a water-soluble sulphate; in fatty acid sulphates;

in the enzymes that contain glutathione and coenzyme A. Sulphur-containing compounds are often prefixed by the term 'thio', derived from the Greek word for sulphur, theion. Thisulphates and thiocyanates are present in body fluids in very small amounts where they are produced in the detoxification of cyanide present in foods, polluted atmospheres and tobacco smoke.

Body content of sulphur resides mainly in keratin, the horny layer of the skin; in fingernails; in toenails; in skin; in the joints. The characteristic smell of burning hair is due to its high sulphur content. The curliness of hair depends upon the sulphur — sulphur bonds of cystine. To straighten hair, these bonds must be opened up. During permanent waving the bonds are opened with one agent then closed again to the desired shape or pattern with another agent. Sheep's wool, which is very curly, can contain 5 per cent of its weight as sulphur.

Food sources of sulphur are (in mg per 100g): mustard powder 1280; dried egg 630; scallops 570; lobster 510; shellfish 250-450; crab 470; nuts 150-380; garlic 370; prawns 370; poultry 200-340; meats 200-330; kidney 170-290; liver 220-270; white fish 200-300; skimmed milk 320; fatty fish 150-260; cheese 230-250; dried peaches 240; roe 240; horseradish 210; offal 140-200; mung beans 190; whole egg 180; Indian tea 180; haricot beans 170; red kidney beans 170; mustard and cress 170; peas 130-180; dried apricots 160; oatmeal 160; wholemeal flour 150; watercress 130; lentils 120; coffee 110; barley 110; wholemeal bread 81. For other foods see individual entries.

Protein supplies most of the sulphur in the diet but some comes in the form of sulphates. A good diet will provide 800mg sulphur daily. Little is known about its intermediate metabolism but excretion parallels that of nitrogen. There is no evidence of any deficiency states in animals or man.

Medicinal uses of sulphur include: a mild laxative when taken orally; a mild antiseptic in ointment form to treat acne; a parasiticide in lotion form, used to treat scabies; with lead acetate to darken grey hair; a depilatory agent to remove body hair.

Medicinal forms include: precipitated sulphur or milk of sulphur, dose 1-4g; sublimed sulphur or flowers of sulphur, dose 1-4g; sulphurated potash, a mixture of potassium polysulphide, potassium sulphite and potassium thiosulphate containing 42 per cent sulphur, used as a lotion on the skin.

---

sultanas, excellent source of potassium, phosphorus and iron with good levels of calcium, magnesium, sulphur and copper. Low sodium food. Sultanas, dried, provide the following minerals (in mg per 100g): sodium 53; potassium 860; calcium 52; magnesium 35; phosphorus 95; iron 1.8; copper 0.35; zinc 0.1; sulphur 44; chloride 16.

---

swedes, low sodium food that provides good levels of potassium, calcium and the trace minerals. In the raw and boiled states respectively, they supply (in mg per 100g): sodium 52, 14; potassium 140, 100; calcium 56, 42; magnesium 11, 7; phosphorus 19, 18; iron 0.4, 0.3; copper 0.05; 0.04; sulphur 39, 31; chloride 31, 9.

---

sweet pickle, a high sodium food that is a good source of potassium, iron and zinc. High sodium and chloride content is due to added salt. It provides the following minerals (in mg per 100g): sodium 1700; potassium 110; calcium 19; magnesium 10; phosphorus 11, iron 2.0; copper 0.10; zinc 1.4; chloride 2600.

---

sweet potatoes, low sodium food that is a rich source of potassium. Provides small quantities of all minerals. Levels for raw and boiled state respectively (in mg per 100g) are: sodium 19, 18; potassium 320, 300; calcium 22, 21; magnesium 13, 12; phosphorus 47, 44; iron 0.7, 0.6; copper 0.16, 0.15; sulphur 16, 15; chloride 64, 60.

---

sweetbread, very good source of trace minerals, sodium and potassium. Rich source of phosphorus and sulphur with moderate levels of calcium and potassium. When fried, supplies the following minerals (in mg per 100g): sodium 210; potassium 260; calcium 34; magnesium 23; phosphorus 420; iron 1.8; copper 0.22; zinc 2.1; sulphur 160; chloride 260.

---

sweet-corn, good source of potassium, magnesium, phosphorus, iron and zinc. Sodium and chloride virtually absent from raw and boiled vegetable but high in canned variety because of added salt. Mineral figures for raw, boiled and canned respectively (in mg per 100g) are: sodium 1, 1, 310; potassium 300, 280, 200; calcium 4, 4, 3; magnesium 46, 45, 23; phosphorus 130, 120, 67; iron 1.1, 0.9, 0.6; copper 0.16, 0.15, 0.05; zinc

1.2, 1.0, 0.6; chloride 11, 14, 460.

---

symptoms of mineral deficiencies in plants, when minerals required by a plant are not in sufficient concentration in a soil or they are prevented from being absorbed by certain factors, specific symptoms appear. Plants in deficient soil may grow but are far from healthy. Typical symptoms are shown in Table 13.

Table 13: Symptoms of mineral deficiencies in plants

Deficient minerals	Symptoms
Nitrogen	Lack of growth and leaves yellowing. Entire plant affected.
Phosphorus	Dark green stunted plants. Delayed maturity. Entire plant affected.
Potassium	Mottled yellowing. Spots of dead areas. Weak stalks. Roots more susceptible to disease.
Sulphur	Yellowing of young leaves. Veins remain green.
Magnesium	Mottled or yellow leaves. Leaf tips turned upwards. Older leaves most affected.
Calcium	Inhibition of root development with death of shoot and root tips. Young leaves and roots most affected.
Iron	Yellowing of veins in young leaves. Stems short and slender. Buds remain alive.
Chlorine	Wilted leaves, yellowing, spots of dead areas. Stunted, thickened roots.
Manganese	Yellow, dead areas between veins. Smallest veins remain green.
Boron	Death of stem. Leaves twisted, pale at base. Swollen, discoloured root tips.
Zinc	Reduction in leaf size. Yellowing. Older leaves most affected.
Copper	Young leaves dark green, twisted, wilted, misshapen.
Molybdenum	Yellowing or twisting and death of young leaves.

T

---

talc, purified, native hydrated magnesium silicate containing a small amount of aluminium silicate. Also known as French chalk. A food additive used as a release agent; as a lubricant in tablet making. Acceptable daily intake is not specified. Permitted as a miscellaneous additive. Excessive inhalation of talc can cause lung disease (pneumoconiosis).

---

tangerines, virtually sodium free, supplying good quantities of potassium and calcium with small amounts of other minerals. Figures for the raw, edible portion (in mg per 100g) are: sodium 2; potassium 160; calcium 42; magnesium 11; phosphorus 17; iron 0.3; copper 0.09; zinc 0.1; sulphur 10; chloride 2.

---

tea, Indian, dried leaf is rich in minerals but infused tea contains only traces of most minerals with high content of manganese (about 1mg per cup). Levels for dried leaf and infusion respectively (in mg per 100g) are: sodium 45, trace; potassium 2160, trace; calcium 430, trace; magnesium 250, 1; phosphorus 630, 1; iron 15.2, trace; copper 1.6, trace; zinc 3.0, trace; sulphur 180 for dried leaf; chloride 52, trace.

---

tetany, a condition resulting from a severe low blood calcium or a reduction in the serum ionized calcium when total blood calcium is normal. It is characterized by sensory symptoms of tingling (pins and needles) of the lips, tongue, fingers and feet; muscular spasms of the hands and feet; spasm and twitching of the face muscles. May be indicative of low body calcium or respiratory or metabolic alkalosis (excess alkali in the body). Treatment is supplementary calcium — orally in mild cases; by intravenous infusion in severe cases.

---

tetrapotassium diphosphate, a food additive that is used as an emulsifying salt, E450a. Acceptable daily intake 373mg per kg body weight. Provides 47.4mg potassium and 18.8mg phosphorus per 100mg. Permitted in some cheeses; in condensed-milk and dried-milk products; as a miscellaneous additive.

---

tetrasodium diphosphate, also known as tetrasodium pyrophosphate. A food additive that functions as a buffer; as an emulsifying salt; as a sequestrant; as a gelling agent; as a stabilizer; E450a. Acceptable daily intake up to 350mg per kg body weight at normal calcium intakes. Provides 34.6mg sodium and 23.3mg phosphorus per 100mg. Permitted in whipping cream; in some cheeses; in condensed-milk and dried-milk products; in boiler feed water for direct steam treatment of milk; as a permitted miscellaneous additive.

---

thyroid, an endocrine gland found in the neck in front of and partially surrounding the thyroid cartilage and the upper end of the trachea.

Term also applies to the thyroid gland of slaughtered animals when it is freed from connective tissue and fat then dried and powdered. Contains not less than 1.70mg and not more than 2.30mg iodine in combination per gram dried gland. One gram dried thyroid equals 5g fresh gland. In man it is used as a source of thyroid hormone in hypothyroidism. In animals it has been used in obesity; kidney failure; chronic skin conditions; and to increase spermatogenesis, libido and milk production.

---

thyrotoxicosis, *see* hyperthyroidism.

---

thyroxine, known also as L-thyroxine; T4. First isolated from thyroid gland by E. C. Kendall of the USA in 1919. It is a natural thyroid hormone containing 4 atoms of iodine per molecule thyroxine. Can also be obtained by chemical synthesis. Used in the treatment of hypothyroidism, particularly for long-term therapy. D-thyroxine has been used to decrease high fat levels in the blood serum. L-thyroxine has been used to treat some cases of obesity. *See* hypothyroidism; iodine; triiodothyronine.

---

tin, chemical symbol Sn, from the Latin *stannum*. Atomic weight 118.7. Occurs in nature as cassiterite, stannite and tealite; abundance in earth's crust is 6mg per kg.

It has been considered to be an essential trace mineral for some animals since the 1960s when rats reared on a tin-free diet were found to have retarded growth. Addition of 1mg tin sulphate to each kg of their diet restored normal growth.

Functions of tin in animals believed to reside in:
1. its stimulating the transcription of RNA and DNA which determine genetic characteristics;
2. protein synthesis through RNA;
3. growth, probably a result of (1) and (2). No functions of tin have been discovered in man.

Food sources of tin are unknown because of difficulty in measurement but canned foods contain higher levels than fresh or frozen foods due to contamination from the container. Even this is reduced because insides of tins are now lacquered. Human diets can provide between 3.5 and 17mg per day, but only when some of the food is of the canned variety. The toxic level is believed to be about 6.0mg per kg body weight so fresh-food diets have a high safety margin. Legal limit of tin in canned foods in 25mg per 100g food. As the toxic amount for a 70kg is 420mg tin, excessive intakes of canned food can approach this level. A concentration of 300mg tin in 100g food causes toxic effects in experimental animals.

Excessive intakes in animals cause anaemia, which can be reversed by feeding extra iron and copper; depressed growth.

Absorption of tin and its salts from the gastrointestinal tract is very poor and most is excreted in the faeces.

Acute toxic effects in man include colic; distension of the abdomen (tympanites or meteorism); constipation.

Chronic toxic effects in man include nausea; colic; headache; weakness; fever; muscle pain; joint pain; tinnitus (head noises).

Inhalation over prolonged periods can cause pneumoconiosis (lung disease). Maximum permissible concentration in atmosphere is 2mg per cubic metre (inorganic tin) or 100μg cubic metre (organic tin).

Medical uses of tin and tin oxide in tablet form include the treatment of boils, carbuncles and acne; tapeworm infestation.

---

tinea versicolor, also known as pityriasis versicolor, a skin infection characterized by multiple patches of lesions varying in colour from white to brown. It is common in young adults. Tan, brown or white, slightly scaling areas are seen on the chest, neck, abdomen and occasionally on the face. These areas do not tan but appear as white 'sun spots'. Treatment is application of undiluted selenium sulphide shampoo or a 2.5 per cent lotion to affected areas (avoiding the scrotum) for 3 or 4 days at bedtime, washing it off in the morning.

---

tissue salts, inorganic mineral salts, specific deficiency of which is believed to be associated with particular diseases. Also known as biochemic tissue salts. Tissue salt therapy is based upon homoeopathic principles first put forward by a German doctor, Wilhelm H. Scheussler of Oldenburg and tested by him from the years 1872 to his death in 1898. Dr Shuessler believed that the disease process was always associated with a deficiency of one or more tissue salts that are normally present, in correct balance, in body tissue cells. By supplying the deficient mineral salts a healthy balance is restored. The twelve tissue salts of Dr Schuessler are: calc. fluor. (calcium fluoride); calc. phos. (calcium phosphate); calc. sulph. (calcium sulphate); ferr. phos. (ferric phosphate or iron phosphate); kali. mur. (potassium chloride); kali. phos. (potassium phosphate); kali. sulph. (potassium sulphate); mag. phos. (magnesium phosphate); nat. mur. (sodium chloride); nat. phos. (sodium phosphate); nat. sulph. (sodium sulphate); silica (silicon dioxide).

True deficiency of a particular mineral is not overcome by sole treatment with a tissue salt, since the quantity in its preparation is minute, based upon homoeopathic principles of dilution. At this dilution the biochemic tissue salt is more likely to influence the way in which the deficient mineral is distributed throughout the body and hence rectify imbalances in that way. Biochemic tissue salts can also influence minerals when they are present in excess in body cells and tissues. Biochemic remedies may therefore be regarded as having a regulatory function on body minerals by influencing the distribution of anions and cations within body cells and in the extracellular fluids bathing those cells.

The preparation of biochemic tissue salts is based upon homoeopathic principles of serial dilution and trituration. One part of the appropriate salt is mixed with nine parts of lactose (milk sugar) and the resultant mixture is vigorously ground and mixed to ensure a completely homogeneous blend. This is termed *trituration* and comprises the first decimal potency called 1X. One part of this potency is mixed with a further nine parts of lactose and the resulting mixture is exhaustively blended to produce the homogeneous second decimal potency 2X. One part of this potency is further diluted with nine parts of lactose in the same manner as before and the resulting mix is termed the third decimal potency 3X. The process, which is known as *serial dilution* (the X simply means that each stage of the dilution is ten-fold) is carried on until the sixth decimal potency. At this stage the tissue salt has been diluted one million times and is known as potency 6X, the most commonly utilized homoeopathic potency. Further dilution to 12X is sometimes carried out but it is seldom necessary to continue beyond this. This constant serial dilution combined with exhaustive blending (trituration) is known as potentization, a term also applied to homoeopathic preparations. The potentized powder is finally highly compressed into small tablets that readily dissolve on or under the tongue.

For best effect the following precautions should be taken:
1. No food or drink should be consumed within 15 minutes of taking a biochemic remedy.
2. Teeth should not be cleaned within the same time restraint.
3. All tissue salts should be kept in containers that will not let in daylight or odours from other substances.
4. Avoid handling the tablets apart from those to be immediately consumed.
5. Transfer to other containers from those in which they are supplied should not be carried out. This is to avoid contamination of the minute amounts of salt left in the biochemic remedy.

The following observations are also important to anyone contemplating biochemic tissue salt remedies:
1. The remedies may be used to treat acute disease (usually infections) and chronic disease (inflammatory and degenerative conditions).
2. Sometimes the condition appears to worsen after taking tissue salts. If it happens during treatment of an acute illness, like an infection, administration of the remedy should cease to allow the body to enter a healing phase. Improvement should then follow. If not, the services of a practitioner, preferably a homoeopathic one, should be sought. Similar considerations apply to treatment of a chronic condition except that worsening may occur several weeks after therapy is initiated. In the same way, therapy should cease to allow the healing phase to come into operation. If necessary when the condition persists, continued therapy at the recommended dose should be re-started.
3. All biochemic tissue salt therapy is safe but those unduly sensitive to lactose should be aware of its presence in these remedies.

4.   No other complementary therapy is affected by tissue salts but the effectiveness of the latter may be reduced and professional advice should be sought.

Properties and applications of the twelve tissue salts are:

Calc. fluor. — calcium fluoride, indicated where tissues have lost their tone, e.g., varicose veins; leg ulcers; eczema; piles; poor blood circulation; constipation; backache; chronic synovitis (arthritis). May be used to treat diseases of the teeth; the bones; the skin; the nails where a surface lesion exists.

Calc. phos. — calcium phosphate, promotes healthy cells in organs and tissues; assists digestion, absorption and assimilation of foodstuffs; improves poor blood circulation; relieves chilblains; relieves generalized pruritus (itching) in the elderly; helps shrink enlarged tonsils and nose polyps. In conjunction with ferr. phos. treats simple anaemia; in alternation with kali. phos. produces more rapid results in relieving pruritus.

Calc. sulph. — calcium sulphate, cleanses the blood and the tissues of the body by removing toxic and waste products. Is used in mild skin conditions; mucous membrane infections; catarrhal complaints where it supplements the action of kali. mur. On its own, calc. sulph. helps relieve head pains and neuralgias in the elderly.

Ferr. phos. — ferric phosphate (or iron phosphate), maintains healthy, strong blood vessel walls; ensures the blood is rich in oxygen to maintain health; complements other treatments for anaemia; relieves congestion, inflammation, high temperature, rapid pulse. Should be given as a standard in the early stage of all acute disorders at frequent intervals. Is an excellent all-round remedy for illnesses associated with ageing and with children. Can be regarded as a first-aid treatment for any sort of muscular or joint injury.

Kali. mur. — potassium chloride, indicated for any soft glandular swelling or those associated with chronic rheumatic conditions. Should be used in conjunction with calc. sulph. which complements its action by purifying the blood. Specific for infantile eczema. When used alternatively with ferr. phos. is particularly beneficial in all children's ailments. Kali. mur. is specific for any sort of thick, white, gelatinous discharges; for a sluggish, underactive liver; for reduced bile production. When alternated with ferr.

phos. it is indicated for inflammatory conditions of the respiratory system like coughs, colds, sore throats, tonsillitis, bronchitis. Problems associated with the digestive system may respond to kali. mur.

Kali. phos. — potassium phosphate, is indicated for mild nerve complaints that cause headaches; dyspepsia; sleeplessness; depression; lethargy; reduced vitality; edginess. Regarded as a general tonic. May also help in nerve-related conditions like shingles (infection of nerve endings with herpes zoster); nervous asthma; nervous insomnia. In these conditions its beneficial action is accentuated by mag. phos. taken in conjunction with it.

Kali. sulph. — potassium sulphate, acts primarily on the skin and mucous membranes of all the internal organs. It treats the feelings of extremes of cold and of heat; pain in the limbs; vague, generalized pains. Any abnormal condition of the skin and mucous membranes, particularly where there is discharge or scaling, will respond to kali. sulph. Specific for catarrh, a condition of the respiratory mucous membranes. Also treats psoriasis of the skin and fungal infections of athlete's foot. In conjunction with silica it restores brittle nails to health; with silica and nat. mur. it helps maintain healthy hair.

Mag. phos. — magnesium phosphate, the anti-spasmodic tissue salt. Like kali. phos. it maintains a healthy nervous system; in conjunction with this tissue salt it relieves cramping, shooting, darting and spasmodic pains. On its own, mag. phos. is indicated for the painful conditions of neuralgia, neuritis, sciatica and headache. Muscular twinges, cramps, hiccoughs, fits of coughing and any sudden, sharp pains will respond to mag. phos. It acts more rapidly when the biochemic salt tablets are taken with a sip of hot water.

Nat. mur. — sodium chloride, restores to normal any part of the system that is too wet or too dry, where water balance is upset. Typical conditions include headache; constipation; hard faeces; soreness of the anus; watery discharge of colds; dry nose and throat; sluggish digestion; thirst, excessive flow of tears and saliva as in neuralgia and toothache; watering eyes; hay fever; respiratory allergies; dryness of the skin; tiredness on waking; craving for salt and salty foods. Nat. mur. stimulates the flow and production of hydrochloric acid in the digestive system. It controls water distribution throughout the body. Has been used to make salt-free or low-salt diets more acceptable to the individual. Relieves insect bites and stings when applied directly to the affected area.

Nat. phos. — sodium phosphate, is an acid neutralizer. Excess acid can give rise to rheumatic conditions; digestive upsets; intestinal disorders; inefficient assimulation of nutrients. Nat. phos. relieves all of these states. It also helps regulate the bile content and flow and so is indicated in the treatment of jaundice, colic, sick headaches and gastric disturbances. It helps promote the absorption of water and so with nat. mur. and nat. sulph. serves to control body-water balance. Nat. phos. helps emulsify fatty acids in the digestive system so it is indicated where fat digestion and absorption is difficult. Specific for relieving gouty and allied conditions due to the deposition of uric acid in the joints. Remedies any condition giving rise to yellow exudates and discharges.

Nat. sulph. — sodium sulphate, controls the density of the extracellular fluids (which bathe the cells) by eliminating excess water. Essential for the healthy functioning of the liver by ensuring an adequate supply of bile to assist in fat digestion. Toxins from body cells are excreted through the cell membrane to the extracellular fluid from where they are eliminated through the kidneys. Nat. sulph. is concerned in this disposal so it is essential to prevent accumulation of toxins in the cells and water. For this reason it is indicated in rheumatic conditions; in biliousness; in treating influenza; in sluggish kidneys; in conditions causing a coated tongue; when there is excess bitterness in the mouth.

Silica — silicon dioxide, acts upon the organic tissues of the body including the bones, joints, glands and skin. It is indicated for any condition where there is pus formation like abscesses, styes and boils. An inflamed throat as in tonsillitis needs biochemic silica. It is also of benefit in nail and hair conditions. Silica restores a healthy skin and normalizes the perspiration. When rheumatic conditions are related to excess uric acid, as in gout, silica functions by dissolving the crystals and excreting them. The mild mental aberrations observed in old people (senile dementia) may respond to silica.

Often a combination of tissue salts is more effective at relieving a variety of related symptoms. Examples are mag. phos., nat. mur., and silica for migraine; ferr. phos., kali. mur., and nat. mur. for coughs, colds and influenza; calc. fluor., calc. phos., kali. phos. and nat. mur. for backache and lumbago; calc. fluor., ferr. phos. and nat. mur. for varicose veins and blood circulation problems; kali. mur., kali. sulph., calc. sulph. and silica for minor skin ailments; ferr. phos., kali. phos. and mag. phos. for sciatica, neuralgia and neuritis; calc. phos., kali. phos. and ferr. phos.

for general debility and nervous exhaustion.

---

titanium dioxide,　a food additive used as a colouring agent, E171. Also known as Pigment White 6. Acceptable daily intake not limited. Provides 60mg titanium per 100mg. Permitted as colouring matter; in specified sugar products; in certain jam products.

---

tomato juice,　very good source of potassium with small amounts of most other minerals present. High sodium and chloride levels are due to added salt. Mineral levels for canned juice (in mg per 100g) are: sodium 230; potassium 260; calcium 10; magnesium 10; phosphorus 20; iron 0.5; copper 0.05; zinc 0.4; chloride 370.

---

tomato purée,　excellent source of all minerals apart from sodium. If brand has added salt, sodium and chloride levels will be increased. It provides the following minerals (in mg per 100g): sodium (for brand without added salt) 20; potassium 1540; calcium 51; magnesium 66; phosphorus 130; iron 5.1; copper 0.63; zinc 1.7; chloride (for brand without added salt) 290.

---

tomato sauce,　good source of potassium with significant quantities of other minerals present. Sodium and chloride levels are high because of added salt. It supplies mineral levels of the following (in mg per 100g): sodium 340; potassium 320; calcium 28; magnesium 14; phosphorus 37; iron 0.7; copper 0.12; zinc 0.4; chloride 560.

---

tomatoes,　very good source of potassium with small but significant amounts of all minerals. Sodium is higher in the canned variety because of added salt. Mineral figures for raw, fried and canned states respectively (in mg per 100g) are: sodium 3, 3, 29; potassium 290, 340, 270; calcium 13, 15, 9; magnesium 11, 13, 11; phosphorus 21, 25, 22; iron 0.4, 0.5, 0.9; copper 0.10, 0.12, 0.11; zinc 0.2, 0.2, 0.3; sulphur 11, 9, not recorded for canned; chloride 51, 59, 78.

---

tongue, excellent source of potassium, phosphorus, iron, copper, zinc and sulphur. Sodium is moderate in the raw meat but is increased in the processed meats available because of added salt. For all varieties, mineral levels vary (in mg per 100g) within the range quoted: sodium 80-1210; potassium 110-300; calcium 6-31; magnesium 13-19; phosphorus 150-230; iron 30-49; copper, 0.37 contained in raw ox pickled variety; zinc, 3.5 contained in raw ox pickled variety; sulphur 190-200; chloride 80-1750.

trace elements, also known as trace minerals. They are elements that occur in the body at very low concentrations, usually less than 0.01 per cent of the body's weight. At least 15 trace elements are presently recognized as essential for warm-blooded animals and birds. They arc, in order of demonstrated need, iron, iodine, copper, manganese, zinc, cobalt, molybdenum, selenium, chromium, tin, vanadium, fluorine, silicon, nickel and arsenic. Man's needs for twelve of them has been demonstrated but it is likely that the other three — arsenic, nickel and tin — are also essential. Difficulty in creating deficiencies of these three in modern diets has been conducive to lack of knowledge of their specific roles in man. All trace elements can also be toxic in man but in most cases the range of intakes between needs and toxicity is wide. Some trace elements are positively harmful in man and these include cadmium, lead and mercury.

Table 14: Recommended daily intakes of selected trace elements

	Age (yrs)	Cu (mg)	Mn (mg)	F (mg)	Cr (μg)	Se (μg)	Mo (μg)
Infants	0-0.5	0.5-0.7	0.5-0.7	0.1-0.5	10-40	10-40	30-60
	0.5-1	0.7-1.0	0.7-1.0	0.2-1.0	20-60	20-60	40-80
Children and	1-3	1.0-1.5	1.0-1.5	0.5-1.5	20-80	20-80	50-100
adolescents	4-6	1.5-2.0	1.5-2.0	1.0-2.5	30-120	30-120	60-150
	7-10	2.0-2.5	2.0-3.0	1.5-2.5	50-200	50-200	100-300
	11+	2.0-3.0	2.5-5.0	1.5-2.5	50-200	50-200	150-500
Adults		2.0-3.0	2.5-5.0	1.5-4.0	50-200	50-200	150-500

(Iodine and iron recommended dietary intakes are quoted in the appropriate entries.)

The functions of trace elements in the body are as integral components of many enzymes and some hormones. Unlike the macro-elements, they play no part in the structure make-up of the body (with the possible exception of fluoride in bones and teeth), nor do they contribute to the electrolyte balance. An excess or a deficiency of trace elements can be wholly or partially responsible for a number of disorders. The toxic trace elements in particular may accumulate in the body and produce ill-effects in an insidious manner.

Estimated safe and adequate daily intakes of selected trace elements have been recommended by the Food and Nutrition Board, National Research Council — National Academy of Sciences, 1980 as shown in Table 14.

---

treacle, a very rich source of potassium, calcium, magnesium, iron and chloride. Moderate levels of sodium, sulphur and copper. Black variety supplies the following mineral levels (in mg per 100g): sodium 96; potassium 1470; calcium 500; magnesium 140; phosphorus 31; iron 9.2; copper 0.43; sulphur 69; chloride 820.

---

triiodothyronine, known also as liothyronine; T3. First isolated from thyroid gland by J. Gross and R. Pitt-Rivers of the UK in 1952. A natural thyroid hormone containing 3 atoms of iodine per molecule triiodothyromine. Can also be obtained by chemical synthesis. Used in the initial therapy of hypothyroidism because it has a faster action and turnover rate than thyroxine.

Elevated blood levels have been found in victims of sudden infant death syndrome. *See* hypothyroidism; iodine; thyroxine.

---

tripe, supplies significant quantities of potassium, calcium, phosphorus, iron, copper and sulphur. Particularly rich in zinc, but has only moderate sodium content. In dressed and stewed form respectively, it supplies the following minerals (in mg per 100g): sodium 46, 73; potassium 8, 100; calcium 75, 150; magnesium 8, 15; phosphorus 37, 90; iron 0.5, 0.7; copper 0.09, 0.14; zinc 1.5, 2.3; sulphur 80, 140; chloride 8, 58.

---

tripotassium citrate, provides 36.2mg potassium in 100mg citrate. Has been used as a supplement; as a mild diuretic; to make the urine less acid; in the treatment of inflammatory conditions of the bladder; to prevent the side-effects of sulphonamide drugs. Has less purgative action than some potassium supplements. Also allowed as a food additive: E332. Usual intake is up to 10g daily in divided doses. Acceptable daily intake is not limited. Used as a buffer; as an emulsifying salt; as a sequestrant. Permitted in sterilized and UHT cream; in some cheeses; in condensed-milk and dried-milk products; in reduced-sugar jam products; as a miscellaneous additive.

---

trisodium citrate, a food additive used as a buffer; as an emulsifying salt; as a sequestrant; as a blood anti-coagulant; E331. Acceptable daily intake not limited. Provides 26.7mg sodium per 100mg. Permitted in sterilized and UHT cream; in some cheeses; in condensed-milk and dried-milk products; in jam and similar products (only for normalizing acidity); as a miscellaneous additive.

---

trisodium orthophosphate, also known as sodium phosphate, tribasic. Used as buffer; as emulsifying salt; as anti-caking agent; E339. Acceptable daily intake up to 350mg per kg body weight at normal calcium intakes. Provides 42.1mg sodium and 18.9mg phosphorus per 100mg. Permitted in sterilized and UHT cream; in some cheeses; in condensed-milk and dried-milk products; boiler feed water for direct steam treatment of milk; as a miscellaneous additive.

---

turkey, very good source of zinc with significant amounts of iron and copper. High in potassium, phosphorus and sulphur. It contains the following range of mineral levels (in mg per 100g): sodium 43-71; potassium 270-340; calcium 6-12; magnesium 19-29; phosphorus 170-230; iron 0.5-1.4; copper 0.11-0.16; zinc 1.2-3.5; sulphur 210-300; chloride 42-62.

---

turnip tops, very good source of calcium and iron. Supplies moderate intakes of potassium, phosphorus, zinc and sulphur. As boiled, provides the following minerals (in mg per 100g): sodium 7; potassium 78; calcium 98; magnesium 10; phosphorus 45; iron 3.1; copper 0.09; zinc 0.4; sulphur 39; chloride 15.

---

turnips, low sodium food that is a good source of calcium and potassium. Mineral levels, in the raw and boiled states respectively (in mg per 100g) are: sodium 58, 28; potassium 240, 160; calcium 59, 55;

magnesium 7, 7; phosphorus 28, 19; iron 0.4, 0.4; copper 0.07, 0.04; sulphur 22, 21; chloride 70, 31.

V

vanadium, chemical symbol V. Atomic weight 50.9. Widely distributed in ores; abundance in earth's crust 100mg per kg.

An essential trace element for rats and chicks, it may also be necessary for human beings. Deficiency in animals causes reduction in red blood cell production leading to anaemia; upset in iron metabolism; lack of growth of bones, teeth and cartilage; increased blood fat levels; increased blood cholesterol levels. It therefore functions in growth; fat metabolism; blood production; and possibly in prevention of dental caries. Feeding vanadium to deficient animals reduces blood fat and cholesterol levels.

Excess vanadium in man may be related to manic depression. Manic-depressives, when fed a low vanadium diet or given extra vitamin C (to remove excess vanadium) showed great improvements as their body levels of vanadium fell. Daily intakes of vanadium in the diet are probably between 100 and 300µg. Most of this passes directly through the system, unabsorbed, but some is retained in the bones and liver.

Food sources are (in µg per 100g): parsley 2950; lobster 1610; radishes 790; dill 460; lettuce 280; gelatin 250; fish bones 240; strawberries 70; whortleberries (bilberries) 54; calf liver 11-51; sardines 46; cucumber 38; apples 33; cauliflower 9; tomatoes 4; potatoes 1. All other foods contain less than 1µg per 100g.

Processed foods may contain more than the fresh variety because of contamination from the vanadium in the stainless steel of processing plants.

Toxic effects have not been reported except the possibility that the trace mineral may be related to manic depression.

vasopressin, also known as anti-diuretic hormone or ADH. A peptide hormone, produced in the pituitary gland, that increases the reabsorption of water by the kidney so preventing excessive losses from the body. Used medically to treat diabetes insipidus.

---

veal, very good source of potassium, phosphorus, sulphur and iron. Sodium present in moderate quantities. When cooked all cuts provide minerals in the range (in mg per 100g) of: sodium 97-110; potassium 360-430; calcium 8-14; magnesium 25-33; phosphorus 260-360; iron 1.2-1.6; sulphur 220-330; chloride 68-120.

---

vermouth, supplies small amounts of all the minerals. Figures for dry and sweet variety respectively (in mg per 100g) are: sodium 17, 28; potassium 40, 30; calcium 7, 6; magnesium 5, 4; phosphorus 7, 6; iron 0.34, 0.36; copper 0.06, 0.04; zinc 0.04, 0.03; chloride 9, 16.

---

vitamin/mineral relationships, functions where each is needed for complete utilization of the other; where both are required for a specific process. Examples are:

1. vitamin D, essential for absorption and assimilation of calcium and phosphate;
2. vitamin C, essential for absorption of iron and its incorporation into haemoglobin;
3. vitamin C, possibly needed for the absorption of calcium phosphate;
4. riboflavin (vitamin B_2), essential for iron utilization in making haemoglobin;
5. vitamin E, complements the action of selenium. Both are present in the enzyme glutathione peroxidase.
6. zinc liberates vitamin A from the liver stores;
7. zinc is essential for absorption of folic acid;
8. calcium is necessary for absorption of vitamin B_{12};
9. zinc and vitamin B_6 are essential and function together in the production of essential brain transmitters;
10. magnesium and vitamin B_6 combine to prevent kidney-stone formation;
11. manganese is needed by intestinal bacteria for synthesis of vitamin K.

W

walnuts,   virtually sodium free and rich in potassium, magnesium, phosphorus, sulphur and the trace elements, iron, copper and zinc. Significant calcium level. Edible portion provides these mineral levels (in mg per 100g): sodium 3; potassium 690; calcium 61; magnesium 130; phosphorus 510; iron 2.4; copper 0.31; zinc 3.0; sulphur 100; chloride 23.

watercress,   rich in calcium, potassium and iron; provides significant quantities of sulphur and chloride. Moderate sodium content. In raw state it supplies the following minerals (in mg per 100g): sodium 60; potassium 310; calcium 220; magnesium 17; phosphorus 52; iron 1.6; copper 0.14; zinc 0.2; sulphur 130; chloride 160.

white cabbage,   rich in potassium but supplies also significant amounts of calcium and the trace elements. Very low in sodium. As raw, it contains the following mineral levels (in mg per 100g): sodium 7; potassium 280; calcium 44; magnesium 13; phosphorus 36; iron 0.4; copper 0.03; zinc 0.3; chloride 23.

white currants,   virtually sodium free. Good levels of potassium with small but significant quantities of other minerals. Levels for raw, stewed without sugar and stewed with sugar respectively (in mg per 100g) are: sodium, identical in all states, 2; potassium 290, 250, 230; calcium 22, 19, 17; magnesium 13, 11, 10; phosphorus 28, 24, 22; iron 0.9, 0.8, 0.7; copper 0.14, 0.12, 0.11; sulphur 24, 21, 19; chloride 11, 9, 9.

white flour,   usually fortified with calcium and iron to provide the following minerals (in mg per 100g): sodium 3; potassium 130; calcium 140; magnesium 36; phosphorus 130; iron 2.2; copper 0.22; zinc 0.9; sulphur 100; chloride 62. Non-fortified provides calcium 15; iron 1.5; with similar levels of other minerals

wholemeal flour, rich in potassium, magnesium and phosphorus and in the trace elements iron, copper and zinc. Significant quantities of all other essential minerals and virtually sodium free. Contains the following mineral levels (in mg per 100g); sodium 3; potassium 360; calcium 35; magnesium 140; phosphorus 340; iron 4.0; copper 0.40; zinc 3.0; chloride 38.

Wilson's disease, hepatolenticular degeneration. A rare familial disease that occurs most often in children whose parents are blood relations. Excessive amounts of copper accumulate in the tissues, due to defective synthesis of caeruloplasmin (which carries copper in blood) in the liver and hence allows copper to be transported in the blood plasma only loosely bound to albumen. Deposition of copper in the liver and brain leads to cirrhosis of the liver and brain disturbances. That in the kidneys causes renal dysfunction. The mineral is also deposited in the eye causing a golden-brown or grey-green pigment ring at the edge of the cornea. Radiating brownish spokes of copper deposits on the lens capsule form the characteristic sunflower cataract.

Treatment is by avoidance of foods high in copper; chelation of the excess copper with chelating drugs such as D-penicillamine or ethylene diamine tetraacetate; displacement of excess copper from the body with zinc.

D-penicillamine can cause acute toxic reactions in about one-third of those treated, e.g., fever, rash, low white blood cell count and low blood platelet count. Vitamin B$_6$ is given at the intake of 25-50mg daily to prevent possible deficiency.

Zinc sulphate, 200 or 300mg three times daily (providing 45 or 68mg elemental zinc three times daily) has also been found to be effective. There were no side-effects.

---

wines, supplies significant quantities of potassium and all the trace elements. Very low in sodium content.

Red wine supplies the following mineral levels (in mg per 100g): sodium 10; potassium 130; calcium 7; magnesium 11; phosphorus 14; iron 0.90; copper 0.12; chloride 18.

Rosé wine provides (in mg per 100g): sodium 4; potassium 75; calcium 12; magnesium 7; phosphorus 6; iron 0.95; copper 0.02; zinc 0.04; chloride 7.

White wine of all varieties (in mg per 100g) provides levels in the range of: sodium 4-21; potassium 57-110; calcium 3-14; magnesium 6-11; phosphorus 6-13; iron 0.50-1.21; copper 0.01-0.05; chloride 4-10.

---

winter cabbage,   good source of potassium and moderate supplier of all other minerals. Virtually sodium free. Mineral levels for raw and boiled respectively (in mg per 100g) are: sodium 7, 4; potassium 390, 160; calcium 57, 38; magnesium 17, 8; phosphorus 54, 34; iron 0.6, 0.4; copper 0.06, 0.03; zinc 0.4, 0.2; chloride 31, 13.

---

wound healing,   needs many micro-nutrients including iron, zinc, vitamins A and C with adequate protein in the diet. The key healing nutrient is zinc which functions in:
1.   rapid cell division, dependent on DNA synthesis, which supplies new cells to close the wound;
2.   the synthesis of collagen which toughens up the newly laid-down cells by meshing these with existing old tissue cells; this process also needs vitamin C;
3.   liberation of vitamin A from the liver; this vitamin is also needed for the rapid rate of production of new tissue cells;
4.   stabilizing cell membranes, keeping them strong and resilient under stress.
   To ensure maximum healing rate, supplementation should provide at least 15mg zinc element daily and possibly double this. Excessive quantities of zinc will not cause faster healing so there is no point in taking more than the recommended supplement.

Y

---

yam,   contains high potassium level with moderate but significant quantities of the other minerals. A low-sodium food. Mineral levels for raw and boiled state respectively (in mg per 100g) are: sodium (not recorded for raw state), boiled 17; potassium 500, 300; calcium 10, 9; magnesium 40, 14; phosphorus 40, 33; iron 0.3, 0.3; copper 0.16, 0.15; zinc 0.4, 0.4;

chloride (not recorded for raw state), 40 for boiled.

---

yeast,   excellent source of all minerals but particularly rich in the trace minerals including chromium and selenium. Torula variety is similar but devoid of chromium and selenium. Mineral quantities for baker's and dried respectively (in mg per 100g) are: sodium 16, 50; potassium 610, 2000; calcium 25, 80; magnesium 59, 230; phosphorus 390, 1290; iron 5.0, 20.0; copper 1.6, 5.0; zinc 2.6, 8.0.

---

yogurt,   excellent source of calcium, potassium, phosphorus and chloride. Small but useful amounts of the trace minerals and only moderate amounts of sodium. Mineral levels vary, according to variety, in the following ranges (in mg per 100g): sodium 64-76; potassium 220-240; calcium 160-180; magnesium 17-20; phosphorus 140; iron 0.09-0.24; copper 0.04-0.10; zinc 0.60-0.69; chloride 150-180.

Z

---

zinc,   chemical symbol Zn. Atomic weight 65.4. Abundance in earth's crust is 0.02 per cent. Occurs in nature as smithsonite (or zinc spar), sphalerite (or zinc blends), zincite, willenite, franklinite and gahnite. Essential trace mineral for plants, animals and human beings.

An adult person contains between 2 and 3g of zinc. Concentration in muscle, liver and kidney is $55\mu g$ per g with other organs containing less. Highest concentrations are in the prostate gland, semen and sperm at levels of 850, 3000 and $2000\mu g$ per g respectively. The eyes contain between 385 and $571\mu g$ per g dry mass. Hair usually contains between 125 and $225\mu g$ per g and reflects the body zinc status of the individual when the hair is growing. In malnutrition hair growth slows down or stops so hair zinc content may not reflect body levels. Sixty-three per cent of body zinc resides in the muscles and bones, with a further 20 per cent in the skin. Blood plasma ranges from 70-120µg zinc per 100ml; red blood cells contain 12-14µg per ml of packed cells while white blood cells may contain 25 times as much. In the blood plasma albumen is the main transport protein for zinc and some reserves of the mineral are bound more firmly to the globulins. There are no specific storage sites known for zinc.

Excretion of zinc is mainly via the faeces and consists of the mineral secreted in the pancreatic and intestinal digestive juices plus that which has not been absorbed from the diet. Urinary excretion is fairly constant and daily losses range from 400-600µg zinc on a normal diet. Starvation results in a marked increase of urinary loss reflecting increased breakdown of body cells. When body levels are low, less is excreted via the urine. Increases in urinary zinc losses occur in porphyria, alcoholism and liver disease and in kidney disease where large amounts of protein are excreted in the urine. Excretion of zinc is increased by diuretic drugs of the thiazide type but decreased by ethacrynic acid or frusemide diuretic drugs. For this reason both types are sometimes given. Sweat losses of zinc may be significant at levels up to 1.0mg per litre but when the mineral is deficient, concentration in the sweat is considerably reduced.

Food content of zinc varies greatly even though it is widely distributed in food stuffs. Foods of animal origin are the best sources and present the zinc in the most easily absorbed form. There is some concern that the zinc content of vegetarian diets may not achieve the recommended intake. A reduction in intake of animal-food products will inevitably lead to a reduction in available dietary zinc. Vegetarian foods with available zinc include carrots, roasted peanuts, canned tomatoes, peas and sweet-corn. Average daily zinc intake of UK citizens calculated from MAFF National Food Survey Committee (1974) was estimated at 11.16mg per day, derived as follows (all figures in mg per day): milk and cream 2.65; eggs 0.27; fats 0.05; sugar and preserves 0; potatoes 0.52; greens 0.22; other green vegetables 0.16; white bread 0.62; brown bread 0.11; others 0.01; flour 0.15; cakes/biscuits 0.18; breakfast cereals 0.30; others 0.28; beverages 0; meat 4.70; fish 0.10; cheese 0.55. Meats, fish and dairy products contributed 8.32mg zinc compared with only 2.84mg from vegetable and cereal sources. The high fibre and phytic acid contents of vegetarian diets may also reduce the availability of zinc when no foods of animal origin are eaten.

Foods rich in zinc are (in mg per 100g): oysters 45-70; liver 7.8; dried brewer's yeast 7.8; shrimps 5.3; crab 5.0; beef 4.3; cheese 4.0; sardines 3.0; canned ham 2.3; wholemeal bread 2.0; eggs 1.5; rye bread 1.3; chicken 1.1; peas 0.7; white bread 0.8; fish 0.4; carrots 0.4; rice 0.35; potatoes 0.29; green beans 0.21; tomatoes 0.2.

Absorption of zinc from diets containing proteins of animal origin (meat, fish, milk, eggs) is more efficient than that from plant products such as cereals and soya beans. The amino acid cysteine helps zinc to be absorbed and animal proteins are rich in this. Factors that are of major importance in giving rise to low zinc availability from the diet are:

1. phytic acid, widely distributed in cereals, mainly legumes and nuts and a few tubers and fruits. It forms highly insoluble metal-phytate complcxcs in the intestine which cannot be absorbed. Significance of effect upon zinc absorption depends on phytate:zinc ratio. With greater ratio than 15, low blood zinc level results; with a ratio of 25 or more growth of the young is significantly impaired.

2. dietary fibre, which contains constituents other than phytic acid that bind zinc strongly in the intestine and prevent its absorption. High intakes of wholegrains, cereals, fruits, vegetables and nuts will supply much dietary fibre. Cooking processes reduce the adverse effects of both phytic acid and dietary fibre on zinc absorption.

3. polyphosphates which are added to many processed foods, particularly frozen and canned meats and fowl, can combine with zinc to form insoluble and hence unavailable zinc phosphates.

4. ethylenediaminetetra-acetate (EDTA) which chelates irreversibly with zinc producing stable, insoluble chelates that immobilize the zinc. EDTA may be introduced during the processing of food.

According to WHO sources, the intakes required to ensure the minimum requirements, taking into account variable availability, are as shown in Table 15.

The estimated requirement whilst breast-feeding is based on a milk content of 5mg per litre and a daily milk secretion of 650ml. Hence the 11.16mg zinc in the average UK diet is adequate for adults but may fall short of requirements for adolescents and pregnant and nursing mothers assuming at least 20 per cent absorption of the dietary mineral. Pregnant and lactating women may make up deficiency by eating more but adolescents on unbalanced diets or with inadequate energy intakes should be supplemented with zinc. In the UK at least 75 per cent of dietary zinc comes from meat, fish, eggs and dairy products, so is highly available. Vegetarians eat more cereal, vegetables and nuts and when dairy products form part of their diet they should receive minimal requirements. Vegans

Table 15: Minimum required intakes of zinc (WHO)

	Age	Retained	Excreted	Total required	mg needed in daily diet at different per cent availability		
					10%	20%	40%
	0- 4 mths	0.35	0.9	1.25	12.5	6.3	3.1
	5-12 mths	0.2	0.9	1.1	11.0	5.5	2.8
Males	1-10 yrs	0.2	1.4	1.6	16.0	8.0	4.0
	11-17 yrs	0.8	2.0	2.8	28.0	14.0	7.0
	18 yrs +	0.2	2.0	2.2	22.0	11.0	5.5
Females	1- 9 yrs	0.15	1.4	1.55	15.5	7.8	3.9
	10-13 yrs	0.65	2.0	2.65	26.5	13.3	6.6
	14-16 yrs	0.2	2.0	2.2	22.0	11.0	5.5
	17 yrs +	0.2	2.0	2.2	22.0	11.0	5.5
Pregnancy	0-20 wks	0.55	2.0	2.55	25.5	12.8	6.4
	21-30 wks	0.9	2.0	2.9	29.0	14.5	7.3
	31-40 wks	1.0	2.0	3.0	30.0	15.0	7.5
Breast feeding		3.45	2.0	5.45	54.5	27.3	13.7

(All figures are in mg zinc.)

who subsist entirely on non-animal foods need to be aware that their diet gives low absorption of zinc that may be further curtailed by high intakes of phytic acid and dietary fibre.

Textured vegetable protein (TVP) diets that are increasingly being used as meat extenders may contribute to lower zinc intakes from the diet. Such products generally contain only one-half or two-thirds the zinc of authentic meat products; in addition they have high phytate:zinc ratios exceeding 25:1. When TVP is the sole source of protein in the diet, low growth rates and decreased blood zinc levels resulted in animal experiments, even when total zinc in the diet was in excess of that recommended. Supplementation with further zinc overcame the problem. These observations illustrate the importance of consuming a varied diet.

Food processing and refining influences the content and availability of zinc for absorption. For example, unrefined rice may contain 1.2mg per 100g; the refined variety provides less than 0.2mg per 100g. Wholewheat flour may contain 3.5mg zinc per 100g; white flour only 0.8mg per 100g. This reduces further in white bread to 0.12mg per 100g. Processing and refining may increase the availability of zinc if the process removes undesirable chelating substances like phytic acid. The addition of complexing agents like EDTA and polyphosphates to food will reduce the amount of zinc available for absorption.

Metabolism of zinc starts with its absorption from the food. Substances in the pancreatic juices, probably amino acids or peptides, bind the zinc and carry it across into the intestinal cells. The same complex is able to exchange the zinc with the plasma epithelial or lining cells of the blood vessels. Here the zinc is held until blood plasma concentrations drop, causing zinc to be released from the plasma epithelial cells and taken up by blood proteins. Hence the entry of zinc into the body is controlled.

Within body cells zinc is complexed with various proteins, peptides and amino acids including numerous enzymes. Some 100 such enzymes are known but those isolated from human tissue are carbonic anhydrase, alcohol dehydrogenase, alkaline phosphatase, lactic dehydrogenase, superoxide dismutase and pancreatic carboxypeptidase. The mineral is also complexed with non-enzyme substances such as nucleic acids.

Interactions of zinc with other minerals include:

1.   that with calcium in the intestinal contents where both minerals combine with phytic acid to produce an insoluble complex;

2.   reaction between zinc and calcium in the bone where zinc is deposited in the soft matrix before mineralization with calcium. Increased deposition of calcium in bone leads to increased uptake of zinc by that bone. When calcium is released from bone as in deficiency, zinc is also released. In these situations zinc may be acting in the enzyme alkaline phosphatase which is needed for the calcification of bone;

3.   that between zinc and copper. When copper is increased in the blood plasma, the uptake of zinc by the plasma proteins from the intestinal cells is impaired and zinc entry into the body is depressed. An increase in the copper:zinc dietary ratio from a normal value of 4 to 14 or 20 causes an increase in blood cholesterol which is potentially important in the development of atherosclerosis. High ratios can be obtained either from increased copper intakes or decreased zinc ones.

4.   antagonism between zinc and cadmium. When both are present in the diet they compete for absorption. High cadmium levels prevent zinc being absorbed and vice versa. Cadmium accumulates in the kidney causing high blood pressure by direct action and by retention of sodium. Zinc in adequate quantity can reverse these effects.

Functions of zinc are:

1.   in growth, where it acts in utilization of nitrogen and sulphur both in production of protein and in the synthesis of DNA. Both DNA and RNA need zinc-containing enzymes for their production and functioning.

Zinc therefore plays a crucial role in the processes of cell division and growth. These may explain the observed growth retardation in zinc-deficient children and impaired rate of wound healing in zinc-deficient adults.

2. in insulin activity, where zinc is needed for release of insulin by the pancreas. Diabetics often have low body zinc levels and excrete the mineral at a greater rate via the kidney than non-diabetics;

3. in releasing vitamin A from its liver stores;

4. in the metabolism of the pituitary gland, the adrenal glands, the ovaries and the testes. Individuals with retarded sexual development and lowered pituitary activity respond to zinc therapy. Zinc is needed for the production of male sperm and of female ova. Lack of zinc causes the testes to atrophy (waste away) and results in failure of ovulation;

5. in the nutrition of the growing foetus. Lack of zinc affects the development of the skeleton, nervous system and brain before birth. Once born, the offspring have learning impairment.

6. in maintaining healthy liver metabolism. Zinc metabolism is deranged in cirrhosis of the liver and in alcoholism. Liver function can be improved with high zinc intakes.

Deficiency states in man give rise to:

1. a clinical syndrome characterized by lack of physical, mental and sexual developments with low plasma zinc levels and a mild anaemia. Occurs in older children and adolescents in poor peasant communities in Egypt, Iran and Turkey where the staple diet is the unleavened bread called tanok. Such bread is high in phytic acid and dietary fibre, both of which inhibit absorption of zinc from the diet. Zinc, which is present in the diet cannot be assimilated. Coupled with this is a very low intake of animal foods with zinc in a usable form. In addition, clay eating is a common practice in these areas and the constituents of clay complex with zinc making it unavailable for absorption. Parasitic diseases cause excessive losses of zinc and a substantial amount of the mineral is lost through sweat. A combination of all these factors produced zinc deficiency in these populations. A change in diet plus zinc supplementation (27mg zinc daily) for several months allowed puberty to develop and growth rates were accelerated.

2. zinc responsive growth failure in young children living in Denver, USA. Despite relative affluence these children ate little meat in their diets and subsisted on 'junk' foods. The diagnosis of zinc deficiency was based on the findings of low hair concentration (less than $70\mu g$ per g), growth failure, impaired sense of taste (hypogeusia), poor appetite and a response to oral zinc treatment;

3. delayed wound healing after surgical or accidental injury. Indolent venous leg ulcers healed more rapidly in those given oral zinc sulphate. The lower the body zinc the greater the rate of healing on zinc treatment. Well-nourished US airmen undergoing minor surgery exhibited more rapid healing when supplemented with zinc.

4. impotence, in men on long-term kidney dialysis. The condition was reversed by adding zinc supplements to the dialysing fluid.

5. acrodermatitis enteropathica, a rare hereditary disease that was once fatal in infancy. Disease appears due to failure of zinc absorption and is treated by injecting the mineral or giving high oral doses. The clinical features are loss of hair, a pustular dermatitis and diarrhoea.

Deficiency has been noted in chronic alcoholism due to increased urinary loss and low food intake; malabsorption due to steatorrhoea, Crohn's disease, ulcerative colitis, coeliac disease, cystic fibrosis; protein-energy malnutrition induced by lack of adequate protein intake; high carbohydrate and low protein diets; long-term kidney dialysis; pancreatic disease; nephrotic syndrome; diabetes mellitus; chronic febrile illness and stress from surgery or burns; post-gastrectomy patients; thalassaemia; sickle-cell anaemia; psoriasis; chronic infections; inflammatory diseases like rheumatoid arthritis; pregnancy; tuberculosis; atherosclerosis; high blood pressure; those who are taking the contraceptive pill; those on high dose or prolonged corticosteroid therapy; Down's syndrome (mongolism); nursing mothers on inadequate intakes of dietary zinc; those with high cadmium intakes.

Symptoms of zinc deficiency are: lesions of the skin similar to eczema especially around the mouth, eyes, vagina, nose and hands; hair loss; diarrhoea; mental apathy; defects in reproductive organs, particularly the testes of the male; decreased growth rate; slow mental development; fatigue; lazy reactions; depression after birth of the infant in the female; lack of maternal instincts; high incidence of congenital abnormalities; loss of sense of smell; loss in appetite; white flecks in the nails; eating of dirt and strange substances by children, known as pica; increased susceptibility to infections.

Therapeutic uses include treatment of skin complaints like acne, eczema, psoriasis and rosacea; prevention and treatment of prostate problems; supplementation in all above conditions where deficiency has been noted; prevention of arteriosclerosis; treatment of certain forms of depression; decreasing fat levels in blood; treatment of acrodermatitis enteropathica; easing the symptoms of a cold by sucking lozenges containing 23mg of zinc as zinc gluconate; supplementation of schizophrenics; supplementation of hyperactive children.

Supplementary forms of zinc are: amino-acid chelated zinc; zinc gluconate; zinc orotate; zinc sulphate.

Recommended daily dietary allowances (RDA) of zinc are published by the Food and Nutrition Board of the USA. They assume a 20 per cent absorption of dietary zinc. The figures are (in mg per day): infants 0-0.5 year, 3.0; 0.5-1.0 year, 5.0; children 1-10 years, 10.0; male and females, 11-51 plus, 15.0. Intakes for pregnant women are 20.0mg; these for nursing mothers are 25.0mg daily. UK and WHO authorities make no recommendations. Canada suggests the following intakes of the mineral (in mg per day): 0-0.5 year, 4.0; 0.5-1.0 year, 5.0; 1-3 years, 5.0; 4-6 years, 6.0; males 7-9 years, 7.0; 10-12 years, 8.0; 13-15 years, 10.0; 16-18 years, 12.0; 19-35 years, 10.0; 36-50 years, 10.0; 51 plus years, 10.0; females 7-9 years, 7.0; 10-12 years, 9.0; 13-15 years, 10.0; 16-18 years, 11.0; 19-35 years, 9.0; 36-50 years, 9.0; 51 plus years, 9.0; pregnant women, 12.0; lactating women, 16.0. Czechoslovak authorities recommend 8mg daily for adults; Danish and Italian authorities recommend 15mg daily for adults.

Toxicity of zinc is low. The range between dietary and therapeutic intakes is wide. Compared with some other minerals like copper, selenium, lead, cadmium and mercury, zinc is non-toxic. Inhalation of zinc fumes by workers in smelting plants and the like represent the vast majority of reported cases. Sometimes poisoning can occur from drinking acidic beverages stored in a zinc-galvanized container. Water from a similar container used in dialysis solutions for a kidney patient has caused acute toxicity characterized by nausea, vomiting and fever.

Doses of zinc sulphate of 220mg three times per day (providing a total daily intake of 150mg zinc) have been used therapeutically without ill-effects. Single doses of 0.6-2.0g zinc sulphate given as a 1 per cent solution may act as an emetic causing mild gastric irritation but no further side-effects. In animals, 0.25mg zinc per g food over many months has been found to cause high blood pressure, but this level exceeds even the highest therapeutic intakes in man.

---

zinc amino-acid chelate, provides 10mg zinc in 100mg. On the basis of animal and clinical studies claimed to be more efficiently absorbed than other zinc supplements. Usual daily dose as supplement is 150-200mg chelate (supplies 15-20mg zinc).

---

zinc gluconate, provides 13mg zinc in 100mg. Supplementary daily dose is 100-150mg (providing 13-19.5mg zinc). Common-cold symptoms relieved by sucking two lozenges, each containing 23mg zinc as zinc gluconate, initially, then one every two wakeful hours for 7 days. Children's dose is one half lozenge every 2 hours, not exceeding six lozenges daily. Zinc gluconate shortened the average duration of common colds by about 7 days. Side-effects or complaints were usually minor and consisted of objectionable taste and mouth irritation, with occasional nausea.

---

zinc orotate, provides 17mg zinc in 100mg. Synthetic derivative, claimed to be better absorbed than zinc salts.

---

zinc sulphate, provides 22.7mg zinc in 100mg (as the heptahydrate). Therapeutic dose is 220mg three times daily (supplies 150mg zinc). Supplementary dose is 220mg daily (supplies 50mg zinc). Large intakes (600mg and above in single dose) may cause gastric irritation leading to vomiting or diarrhoea.

BIBLIOGRAPHY

Comprehensive Biochemistry, vol 21, Metabolism of Vitamins and Trace Elements, Ed. Florkin & Stotz Pub. by Elsevier Publishing Co., Amsterdam, 1970.

Handbook of Geriatric Nutrition, Ed. by Jeng M. Hsu & Robert L. Davis. Pub. by Noyes Publications N.J., U.S.A., 1981.

Heavy Metal Toxicity & Safety, T. D. Luckey, B. Veningopal & D. Hutchinson. Pub. by Georg Thieme, Stuttgart, 1975.

Human Nutrition & Dietetics, 7th Edition, S. Davidson, R. Passmore, J. F. Brock, A. D. Truswell. Pub. by Churchill Livingstone, Edinburgh, London and New York, 1979.

Martindale the Extra Pharmacopoeia, 28th Edition. Pub. by Pharmaceutical Press, London, 1982.

Mental and Elemental Nutrients, Carl J. Pfieffer. Pub. by Keats Publishing Inc., New Carrean, Conn., U.S.A., 1975.

Minerals and Your Health, L. Mervyn. Pub. by George, Allen and Unwin, London, 1980.

Nutrition and Killer Diseases, Edition by John Rose. Pub. by Noyes Publications, N.J., U.S.A., 1982.

The Complete Book of Minerals for Health. Pub. by Rodale Press, Penn., U.S.A., 1981.

The Composition of Foods, A. A. Paul & A. T. Southgate, HMSO, London 4th Edition, 1978.

The Trace Elements and Man, Henry A. Shroeder. Pub. by The Devin-Adair Co., Conn., U.S.A., 1982.

Trace Elements in Human and Animal Nutrition, E. J. Underwood. Pub. by Academic Press, London, 1977.

Trace Elements in Human Health and Disease, Volumes 1 and 2. Ed. by A. S. Prasad. Pub. by Academic Press Inc., New York, San Francisco, London, 1976.